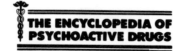

THE ENCYCLOPEDIA OF PSYCHOACTIVE DRUGS

IN 25 VOLUMES
Each title on a specific drug or drug-related problem

INHALANTS

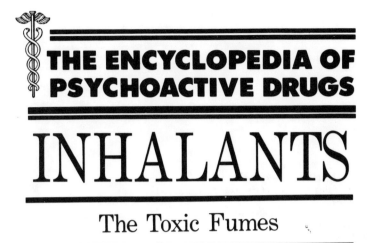

THE ENCYCLOPEDIA OF PSYCHOACTIVE DRUGS

INHALANTS

The Toxic Fumes

JOHN R. GLOWA, Ph.D.

Clinical Neurosciences Branch
National Institute of Mental Health

1986
CHELSEA HOUSE PUBLISHERS
NEW YORK
NEW HAVEN   PHILADELPHIA

SENIOR EDITOR: William P. Hansen
ASSOCIATE EDITORS: John Haney, Richard S. Mandell
ASSISTANT EDITORS: Paula Edelson, Perry Scott King
CAPTIONS: Ian Ensign
EDITORIAL COORDINATOR: Karyn Gullen Browne
ART DIRECTOR: Susan Lusk
LAYOUT: Carol McDougall
ART ASSISTANTS: Victoria Tomaselli
       Noreen M. Lamb
PICTURE RESEARCH: Ian Ensign

First Printing

Library of Congress Cataloging-in-Publication Data
Glowa, John R.
  Inhalants: the toxic fumes
  (The Encyclopedia of psychoactive drugs)
  Bibliography: p.
  Includes index.
  Summary: Examines the use of volatile hydrocarbons
such as paint thinners, glue, and cleaning fluid as
inhalants, a rapidly-growing form of drug abuse.
  1. Substance abuse—Juvenile literature. 2. Youth—
Substance use—Juvenile literature. [1. Drug abuse]
I. Title. II. Series.
RC564.G55 1986   616.86′4   85-32569

ISBN 0-87754-758-0

Chelsea House Publishers
Harold Steinberg, Chairman & Publisher
Susan Lusk, Vice President
A Division of Chelsea House Educational Communications, Inc.

133 Christopher Street, New York, NY 10014

345 Whitney Avenue, New Haven, CT 05510

5014 West Chester Pike, Edgemont, PA 19028

Photos courtesy of AP/Wide World Photos, Art Resource, Peter Furst, New York
Academy of Medicine, New York Public Library, UPI/Bettmann Newsphotos, The
Washington Post.

CONTENTS

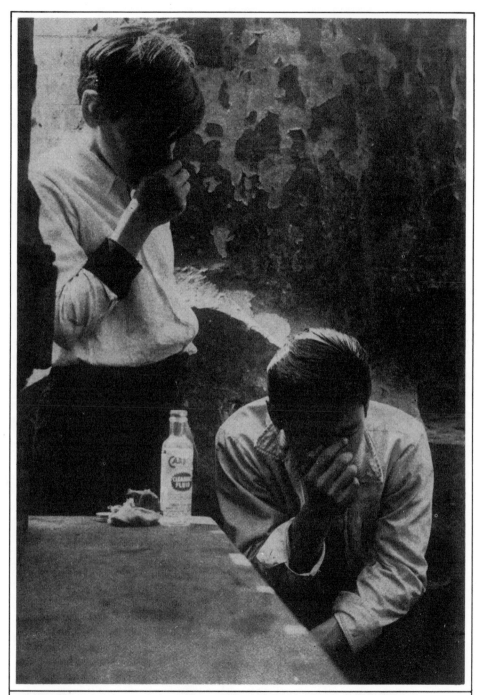

Two adolescents getting high by inhaling the fumes from a household cleaning fluid. Because of the easy availability of volatile solvents, the use of inhalants has become a widespread and dangerous problem.

FOREWORD

In the Mainstream of American Life

The rapid growth of drug use and abuse is one of the most dramatic changes in the fabric of American society in the last 20 years. The United States has the highest level of psychoactive drug use of any industrialized society. It is 10 to 30 times greater than it was 20 years ago.

According to a recent Gallup poll, young people consider drugs the leading problem that they face. One of the legacies of the social upheaval of the 1960s is that psychoactive drugs have become part of the mainstream of American life. Schools, homes, and communities cannot be "drug proofed." There is a demand for drugs—and the supply is plentiful. Social norms have changed and drugs are not only available—they are everywhere.

Almost all drug use begins in the preteen and teenage years. These years are few in the total life cycle, but critical in the maturation process. During these years adolescents face the difficult tasks of discovering their identity, clarifying their sexual roles, asserting their independence, learning to cope with authority, and searching for goals that will give their lives meaning. During this intense period of growth, conflict is inevitable and the temptation to use drugs is great. Drugs are readily available, adolescents are curious and vulnerable, there is peer pressure to experiment, and there is the temptation to escape from conflicts.

No matter what their age or socioeconomic status, no group is immune to the allure and effects of psychoactive drugs. The U.S. Surgeon General's report, "Healthy People," indicates that 30% of all deaths in the United States

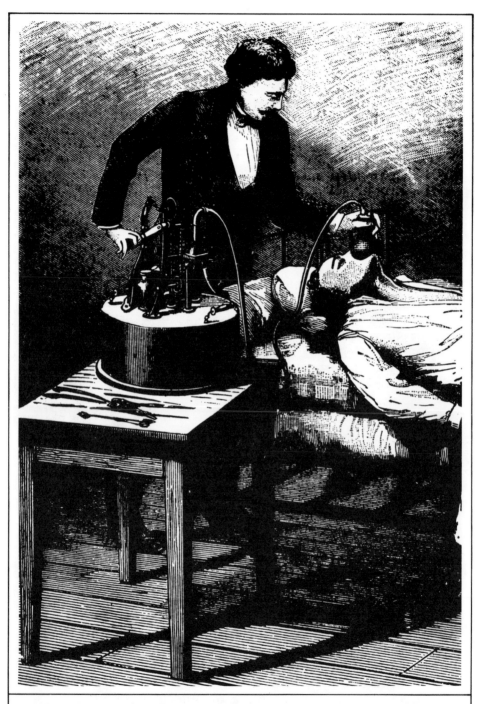

A 19th-century woodcut shows a surgeon using a crude pump to administer ether to a patient. Ether was first used as an anesthetic in the 1840s.

are premature because of alcohol and tobacco use. However, the most shocking development in this report is that mortality in the age group between 15 and 24 has increased since 1960 despite the fact that death rates for all other age groups have declined in the 20th century. Accidents, suicides, and homicides are the leading cause of death in young people 15 to 24 years of age. In many cases the deaths are directly related to drug use.

THE ENCYCLOPEDIA OF PSYCHOACTIVE DRUGS answers the questions that young people are likely to ask about drugs, as well as those they might not think to ask, but should. Topics include: what it means to be intoxicated; how drugs affect mood; why people take drugs; who takes them; when they take them; and how much they take. They will learn what happens to a drug when it enters the body. They will learn what it means to get "hooked" and how it happens. They will learn how drugs affect their driving, their schoolwork, and those around them—their peers, their family, their friends, and their employers. They will learn what the signs are that indicate that a friend or a family member may have a drug problem and to identify four stages leading from drug use to drug abuse. Myths about drugs are dispelled.

National surveys indicate that students are eager for information about drugs and that they respond to it. Students not only need information about drugs—they want information. How they get it often proves crucial. Providing young people with accurate knowledge about drugs is one of the most critical aspects.

THE ENCYCLOPEDIA OF PSYCHOACTIVE DRUGS synthesizes the wealth of new information in this field and demystifies this complex and important subject. Each volume in the series is written by an expert in the field. Handsomely illustrated, this multi-volume series is geared for teenage readers. Young people will read these books, share them, talk about them, and make more informed decisions because of them.

Miriam Cohen, Ph.D.
Contributing Editor

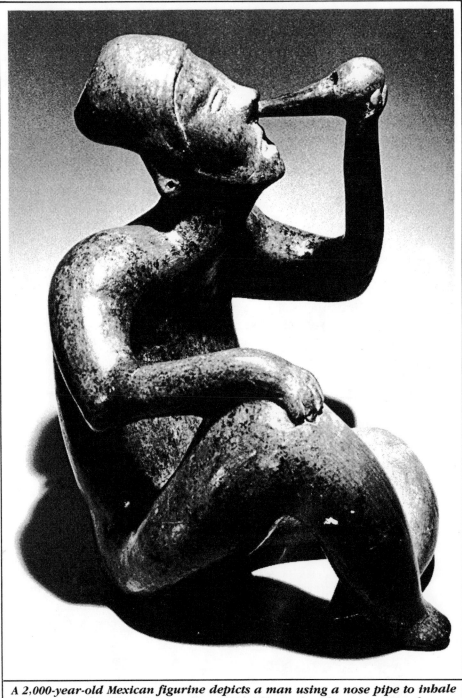

A 2,000-year-old Mexican figurine depicts a man using a nose pipe to inhale psychoactive snuff. Artifacts such as this indicate that the properties of inhaled substances have been known for centuries.

INTRODUCTION

The Gift of Wizardry
Use and Abuse

JACK H. MENDELSON, M.D.
NANCY K. MELLO, PH.D.
Alcohol and Drug Abuse Research Center
Harvard Medical School—McLean Hospital

Dorothy to the Wizard:

"I think you are a very bad man," said Dorothy.
"Oh, no, my dear; I'm really a very good man; but I'm a very bad Wizard."

—from THE WIZARD OF OZ

Man is endowed with the gift of wizardry, a talent for discovery and invention. The discovery and invention of substances that change the way we feel and behave are among man's special accomplishments, and like so many other products of our wizardry, these substances have the capacity to harm as well as to help. The substance itself is neutral, an intricate molecular structure. Yet, "too much" can be sickening, even deadly. It is man who decides how each substance is used, and it is man's beliefs and perceptions that give this neutral substance the attributes to heal or destroy.

Consider alcohol—available to all and yet regarded with intense ambivalence from biblical times to the present day. The use of alcoholic beverages dates back to our earliest ancestors. Alcohol use and misuse became associated with the worship of gods and demons. One of the most powerful Greek gods was Dionysus, lord of fruitfulness and god of wine. The Romans adopted Dionysus but changed his name to Bacchus. Festivals and holidays associated with Bacchus celebrated the harvest and the origins of life. Time has blurred the images of the Bacchanalian festival, but the theme of drunkenness as a major part of celebration has survived the pagan gods and remains a familiar part of modern society. The term "Bacchanalian festival" conveys a more appealing image than "drunken orgy" or "pot party," but whatever the label, some of the celebrants will inevitably start up the "high" escalator to the next plateau. Once there, the de-escalation is difficult for many.

According to reliable estimates, one out of every ten Americans develops a serious alcohol-related problem sometime in his or her lifetime. In addition, automobile accidents caused by drunken drivers claim the lives of tens of thousands every year. Many of the victims are gifted young people, just starting out in adult life. Hospital emergency rooms abound with patients seeking help for alcohol-related injuries.

Who is to blame? Can we blame the many manufacturers who produce such an amazing variety of alcoholic beverages? Should we blame the educators who fail to explain the perils of intoxication, or so exaggerate the dangers of drinking that no one could possibly believe them? Are friends to blame— those peers who urge others to "drink more and faster," or the macho types who stress the importance of being able to "hold your liquor"? Casting blame, however, is hardly constructive, and pointing the finger is a fruitless way to deal with problems. Alcoholism and drug abuse have few culprits but many victims. Accountability begins with each of us, every time we choose to use or to misuse an intoxicating substance.

It is ironic that some of man's earliest medicines, derived from natural plant products, are used today to poison and to intoxicate. Relief from pain and suffering is one of society's many continuing goals. Over 3,000 years ago, the Therapeutic Papyrus of Thebes, one of our earliest written records, gave instructions for the use of opium in the treatment of pain. Opium, in the form of its major derivative, morphine, remains one of the most powerful drugs we have for pain relief. But opium, morphine, and similar compounds, such as heroin, have also been used by many to induce changes in mood and feeling. Another example of man's misuse of a natural substance is the coca leaf, which for centuries was used by the Indians of Peru to reduce fatigue and hunger. Its modern derivative, cocaine, has important medical use as a local anesthetic. Unfortunately, its increasing abuse in the 1980s has reached epidemic proportions.

The purpose of this series is to provide information about the nature and behavioral effects of alcohol and drugs, and the probable consequences of their use. The information presented here (and in other books in this series) is based on many clinical and laboratory studies and observations by people from diverse walks of life.

Over the centuries, novelists, poets, and dramatists have provided us with many insights into the beneficial and problematic aspects of alcohol and drug use. Physicians, lawyers, biologists, psychologists, and social scientists have contributed to a better understanding of the causes and consequences of using these substances. The authors in this series have attempted to gather and condense all the latest information about drug use and abuse. They have also described the sometimes wide gaps in our knowledge and have suggested some new ways to answer many difficult questions.

One such question, for example, is how do alcohol and drug problems get started? And what is the best way to treat them when they do? Not too many years ago, alcoholics and drug abusers were regarded as evil, immoral, or both. It is now recognized that these persons suffer from very complicated diseases involving complex biological, psychological, and social problems. To understand how the disease begins and progresses, it is necessary to understand the nature of the substance, the behavior and genetic makeup of the afflicted person, and the characteristics of the society or culture in which he lives.

The diagram below shows the interaction of these three factors. The arrows indicate that the substance not only affects the user personally, but the society as well. Society influences attitudes towards the substance, which in turn affect its availability. The substance's impact upon the society may support or discourage the use and abuse of that substance.

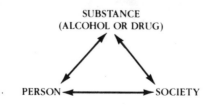

SUBSTANCE
(ALCOHOL OR DRUG)

PERSON — SOCIETY

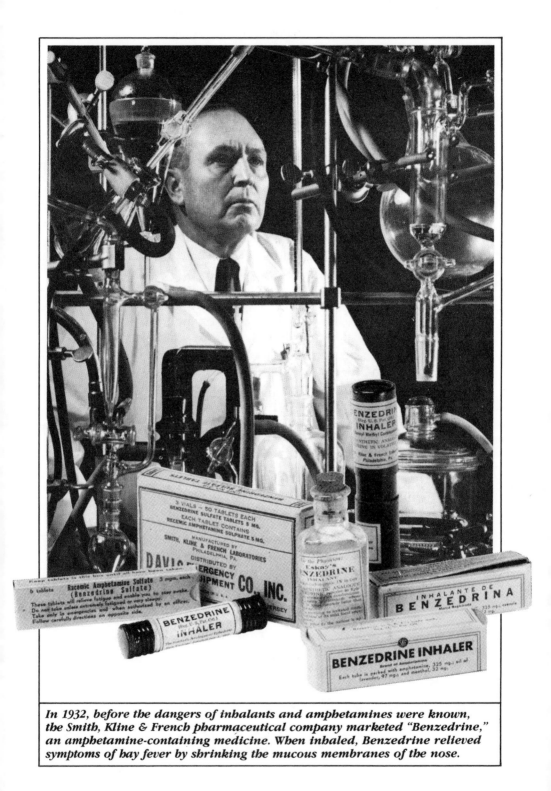

In 1932, before the dangers of inhalants and amphetamines were known, the Smith, Kline & French pharmaceutical company marketed "Benzedrine," an amphetamine-containing medicine. When inhaled, Benzedrine relieved symptoms of hay fever by shrinking the mucous membranes of the nose.

Although many of the social environments we live in are very similar, some of the most subtle differences can strongly influence our thinking and behavior. Where we live, go to school and work, whom we discuss things with—all influence our opinions about drug use and misuse. Yet we also share certain commonly accepted beliefs that outweigh any differences in our attitudes. The authors in this series have tried to identify and discuss the central, most crucial issues concerning drug use and misuse.

Regrettably, man's wizardry in developing new substances in medical therapeutics has not always been paralleled by intelligent usage. Although we do know a great deal about the effects of alcohol and drugs, we have yet to learn how to impart that knowledge, especially to young adults.

Does it matter? What harm does it do to smoke a little pot or have a few beers? What is it like to be intoxicated? How long does it last? Will it make me feel really fine? Will it make me sick? What are the risks? These are but a few of the questions answered in this series, which, hopefully, will enable the reader to make wise decisions concerning the crucial issue of drugs.

Information sensibly acted upon can go a long way towards helping everyone develop his or her best self. As one keen and sensitive observer, Dr. Lewis Thomas, has said,

> There is nothing at all absurd about the human condition. We matter. It seems to me a good guess, hazarded by a good many people who have thought about it, that we may be engaged in the formation of something like a mind for the life of this planet. If this is so, we are still at the most primitive stage, still fumbling with language and thinking, but infinitely capacitated for the future. Looked at this way, it is remarkable that we've come as far as we have in so short a period, really no time at all as geologists measure time. We are the newest, the youngest, and the brightest thing around.

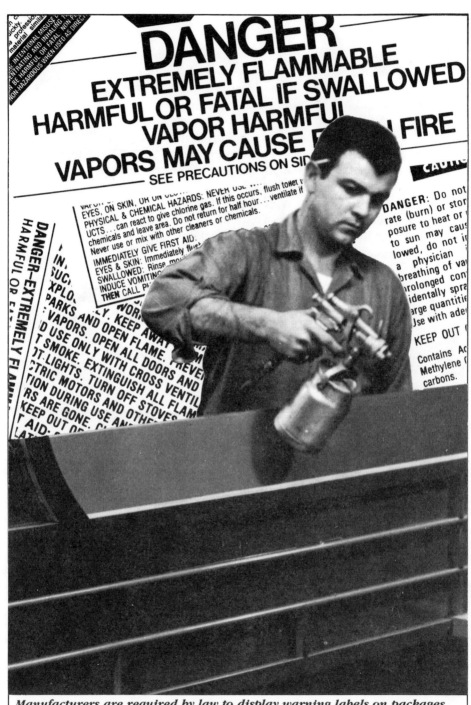

Manufacturers are required by law to display warning labels on packages of thinners, glues, and solvents. One should consider these warnings carefully before entertaining the idea of misusing such products.

AUTHOR'S PREFACE

Inhalants are substances that are sniffed in order to produce mind-altering and/or behavioral effects. Although people inhale many drugs, including nicotine, cocaine, PCP (angel dust), and marijuana, to achieve similar effects, inhalants belong to a different class of drugs because of their chemical structure, their method of consumption, and their unique effects. Most inhalants are part of a large, but not very well-known, group of chemicals called *volatile organic solvents*. One example of such a substance is toluene, a chemical that manufacturers previously included in glue. Toluene was frequently abused when glue-sniffing was popular in the 1970s. People continue to inhale chemical substances, though this is probably the least well-known form of drug abuse today.

In many ways, solvent abuse is similar to other forms of drug abuse, including alcoholism. For example, initially the abuser may sniff only occasionally, either alone or in social settings. But as inhalant use becomes more frequent, the person often becomes compulsive and gradually loses control over the ability to stop sniffing. Each day the user consumes larger amounts of the solvent and often he or she begins to hide the habit from others. Over time no one, not even the drug abuser, is aware of the extent to which drug use has become compulsive. This behavior can lead to tragic consequences.

In one case of solvent abuse, a young German girl was attracted to the smell of an organic solvent known as *trichloroethylene*, a common cleaning compound. She frequently sniffed the solvent until one day her father found her asleep in the bathroom. After warning her about the dangers of sniffing this substance, he locked the cleaner in a cabinet. However, the key to the girl's bureau also unlocked this cabinet, and she was able to continue the sniffing without her parents' knowledge. Several months later she died after inhaling a lethal amount of the solvent. Although death due to solvent abuse is not uncommon, excessive solvent use more often leads to a psychotic-like episode.

Solvent abuse is growing, and few people are aware of this development. More people regularly use volatile organic solvents, such as alcohol and gasoline, than any substance from the other major classes of drugs, including LSD or heroin. There is growing evidence to suggest that solvent abuse often begins at an early age and is often followed by experimentation with and subsequent use of many different drugs such as hallucinogens or opiates. Because volatile organic solvents are readily available, quite inexpensive, and easily concealed, they have a very high abuse potential. This book will focus on the nature of solvent use and attempt to identify the factors related to solvent abuse.

There are many different types of solvents, some of whose effects have not yet been identified. Figure 2 shows the chemical structures of some common forms. Both aliphatic and aromatic hydrocarbons have only carbon and hydrogen atoms. Aliphatic hydrocarbons are composed of an open chain of carbon atoms, and aromatic hydrocarbons, given this name because of their distinctive odors, are made up of rings of carbon atoms. Unlike these pure hydrocarbons, many other organic solvents have additional elements, such as oxygen, chlorine, and nitrogen, that influence the effects of the compound. Some subclasses of solvents are defined by the bonds these elements make with the carbon atoms. Ketones, alcohols, and halogenated hydrocarbons are examples of subclasses. Many solvents consist of a combination of these subclasses. Paint thinner, for instance, is a mixture of toluene, acetone, and methanol.

There are many theories of how volatile organic solvents act on the body. However, the definition of each of the three words that make up the name of these substances form the basis of all explanations. A volatile substance is one that is usually a liquid, although it will boil, or become a vapor, under normal conditions at room temperature. In a gaseous state a substance is readily absorbed through the lungs and into the bloodstream, in which it very rapidly travels to the brain. The amount of liquid that is vaporized—one factor that determines how great an effect an inhalant will have—is related to the drug's particular chemical properties. Less volatile solvents, such as most of the alcohols, are not usually inhaled. Most inhalants, however, do readily volatilize and thus are easy to inhale. Therefore, they have a high abuse potential.

Most solvents are organic, which means they belong to a family of chemicals that contain carbon. Part of the reason these solvents are able to interact with bodily functions is that all living organisms are also organic and thus share certain qualities. (This theory and additional ones that attempt to explain the mechanism of action of volatile organic solvents are discussed in Chapter 2.)

Solvents are substances that dissolve or mix with other less soluble compounds and often pass readily into the body, sometimes even if just placed on the skin. There is evidence to suggest that once in the body volatile organic solvents uniquely affect tissues, such as the brain, that are rich in lipids, or fats. Solvents may produce their behavioral effects by dissolving nerve tissue membranes in the brain, thereby changing their normal functioning. In fact, for many years this has been the popular theory of how anesthetics produce their effects. However, not all inhalants work in this manner.

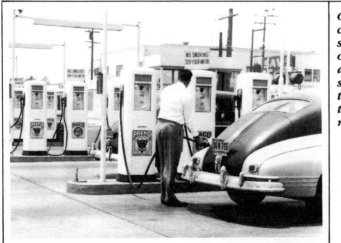

Gasoline is a common volatile solvent. Inhalation of its fumes causes dizziness as well as serious damage to the blood vessels of the brain and respiratory system.

Solvents are ingested, distributed, and eliminated from the body in ways that depend upon the type of solvent and the way in which a person is exposed to it (see Chapter 3). Although most solvents are sniffed, or inhaled, other routes of administration are occasionally used. To evaluate the effects of any drug one must take into consideration how the drug enters the body. This is because both the positive and negative effects are determined by which systems of the body (circulatory, nervous, and gastrointestinal, for example) come into contact with and are affected by the drug. Patterns of intake are also important. For example, factory workers are often exposed to volatile organic solvents at the workplace and inadvertently develop a dependency on them. Because of this initial, accidental contact, these individuals may later seek out these substances and indulge in solvent abuse.

With prolonged exposure, the effects of inhalants sometimes lessen. Occasionally, however, the reverse is true, and the initial effect may be so overwhelming that it results in a permanent aversion to the substance. Thus, the type of exposure influences both the effect of the inhalant and the degree to which it is dangerous.

Recently, scientists have designed experiments that use animals to study indirectly the effects of inhalants on humans (see Chapter 4). Because animals such as rats and monkeys will work to obtain solvents, it is possible to use these animals to identify those substances with high abuse potential and to

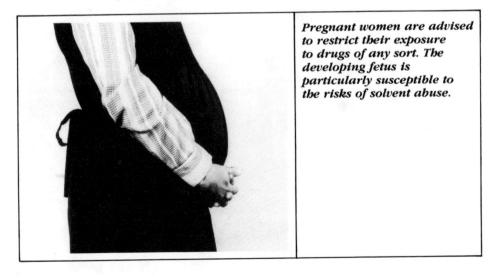

Pregnant women are advised to restrict their exposure to drugs of any sort. The developing fetus is particularly susceptible to the risks of solvent abuse.

develop methods for discouraging solvent abuse. Similar experimental methods can also be used to evaluate the harmful
effects of these chemicals and the acquired data can provide
the necessary evidence for removing the truly dangerous
solvents from the workplace.

Volatile organic solvents produce more unwanted and/
or toxic effects than do most other drugs (see Chapter 5).
Some of these toxic effects are reversible, but others, such
as blindness, are not. Even very brief exposures can disrupt
the normal function of the heart, sometimes even causing
death. Single exposures can disrupt normal brain activity and
lead to the destruction of brain cells. Also, exposure early in
pregnancy is very likely to have adverse effects on the normal
patterns of development of the growing embryo.

Clearly, people may be exposing themselves to considerable risk by abusing solvents. Recent studies have shown
that several factors associated with the chronic solvent abuser
relate to both the individual and the environment in which
he or she lives (see Chapter 6). Solvent abuse is influenced
by peer pressure, availability, cost, and the prevalence of
solvent abuse in the population. In general, solvent abuse is
more common among the lower socioeconomic populations.
One of the many possible reasons for this is that, in general,
these substances are readily available and inexpensive. For
example, the current price of a gallon of gasoline allows a
person to purchase enough volatile organic solvent to last
several days.

On the other hand, if these substances are so cheap, and
if their effects are so pleasurable, why are they not used by
more people? Some of the answers to this question depend
on the social consequences of solvent abuse, or how one's
family and friends feel about this practice.

Since volatile organic solvents are dangerous to use, it
is perhaps surprising that extensive efforts have not been
made to curb their abuse. The reason little control currently
exists seems to be related to the lack of knowledge regarding
the prevalence of solvent abuse and the lack of information
concerning the dangers. As there are grave medical, psychological, and sociological consequences of sniffing, both the
individual abuser and those who live in a community where
abuse exists need to educate themselves on the hazards of
these substances.

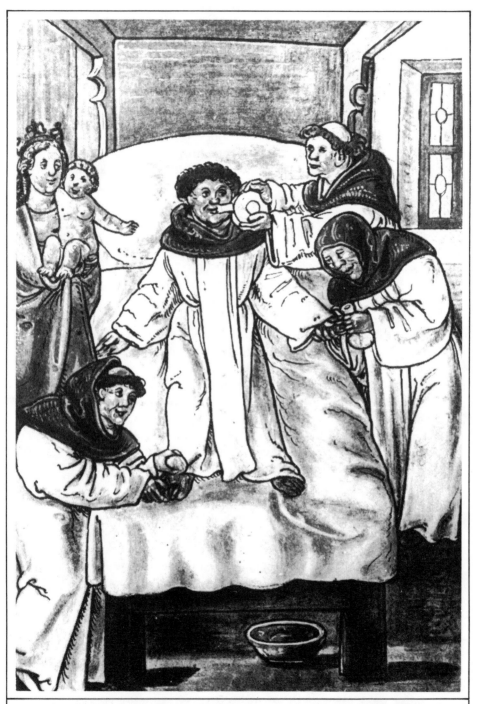

An early 16th-century painting depicts a monk inhaling alcoholic fumes from a flask in an attempt to induce anesthesia.

CHAPTER 1

THE HISTORY OF SOLVENTS

*T*hroughout all of recorded history, people have inhaled drugs to experience their potent effects. At the oracle of Delphi in ancient Greece, one of the mediums, a female priestess known as Pythoness, would sit over a fire in which laurel leaves were burning. The high concentration of carbon dioxide produced during combustion was sufficient to induce in her an ecstatic, mind-altering experience. In this state she was believed to be the mouthpiece of the resident deity, and she would utter prophetic observations that were interpreted and used by those who gathered around her.

In Biblical Palestine and ancient Egypt, ointments and perfumes were freely used to enhance religious worship. Archeologists have unearthed stone altars from the ancient Mesopotamian city of Babylon and from Palestine that were used to burn incense made of aromatic woods and spices. In many or most cases these seemingly innocent substances were, in fact, psychoactive drugs. In the Mediterranean islands 2,500 years ago and in Africa hundreds of years ago, marijuana leaves and flowers were thrown into fires and the smoke was inhaled. During religious ceremonies the North and South American Indians often inhaled hallucinogenic substances.

In actuality, many substances, such as tobacco and opium, will produce effects when they are smoked and/or inhaled. Some of these effects can be attributed to *anoxia*, or a lack of oxygen, resulting from the combination of holding one's breath and the body's absorption of high concentrations of carbon dioxide in the smoke. Though the degree to which anoxia contributes to the physiological and/or psychological effects of most solvents is unknown, for inhalants such as nitrous oxide (N_2O), at least part of the euphoria is related to oxygen deprivation.

Ethanol Drinking

The first known instance of solvent abuse was ethanol drinking. Ethanol, the type of alcohol found in beer, wine, and hard liquors, is produced by the fermentation of sugars in fruits and grains. Fermentation is a chemical process by which yeast consumes sugars and produces effervescence and alcohol. The amount of sugar in the fruit or grain is directly related to the concentration of ethanol—the higher the sugar content, the greater the alcohol concentration. However, as the concentration rises to about 14%, the alcohol kills the yeast and the fermentation process stops. Thus, beer and wine rarely have more than 14% alcohol. The concentration of alcohol can be increased by distilling, or boiling off, the al-

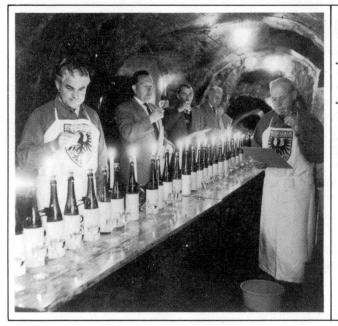

Winemasters in the cellar of a German winery testing wine for taste, body, color, and bouquet. The solvent ethanol, found in wine, beer, and hard liquors, is intoxicating when drunk but does not have strong effects when inhaled.

cohol and collecting it. Distillation, used to produce beverages such as vodka and gin, can produce almost pure alcohol, but even at this concentration the ethanol is not volatile enough to produce profound effects when sniffed. Therefore, though brandy sniffing can result in the inhalation of ethanol, this type of liqueur is typically consumed as a beverage.

Chloroform

As more volatile agents were produced, people began to notice that inhaling these agents produced profound behavioral effects. In 1831 chloroform was discovered independently and simultaneously in Germany, France, and the United States. Accounts of its abuse in the United States were reported the same year. Dentist Horace Wills, the first person in the United States to use nitrous oxide in surgery, died from complications resulting from his own chronic chloroform abuse.

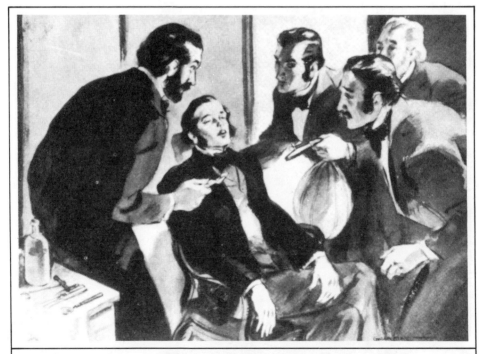

A watercolor depicts the incident where Horace Wells, after inhaling nitrous oxide, felt no pain when his tooth was extracted.

The paper by American researcher Samuel Guthrie that reported his discovery of chloroform clearly illustrates the feelings that were to persist for many years:

A great number of persons have drunk of the solution ... in my laboratory, not very freely, but frequently to the point of intoxication, and so far as I have observed, it has appeared to be singularly grateful, both to the palate and stomach, producing a lively flow of animal spirits, and consequent loquacity; and leaving, after its operation, little of that depression consequent upon the use of ardent spirits [alcohol].

In Scotland in 1847 Dr. James Y. Simpson introduced chloroform for its use as an anesthetic during surgery and childbirth. However, clergymen were opposed to its obstetrical use and cited God's word in Genesis 3:15 as their definitive defense: "In pain you shall bring forth children." Simpson, however, was also able to refer to the Bible to illustrate how even God had used an anesthetic while re-

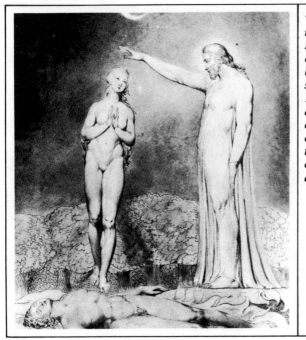

"The Creation of Eve," a watercolor by William Blake, depicts the Biblical episode in which God brings Eve out of a sleeping Adam's side. In 1847 Dr. James Simpson, an early anesthesiologist, cited this passage to convince the church to allow the anesthetic use of chloroform during surgery.

moving Adam's rib to create Eve: "So the Lord God caused a deep sleep to fall upon the man, and while he slept took one of his ribs...." The clergy conceded, and chloroform became so popular that Queen Victoria knighted Dr. Simpson after he delivered her eighth child. However, as other anesthetics were accepted and the number of reported overdoses increased, its popularity declined.

Nitrous Oxide

Nitrous oxide (N_2O) was discovered in 1776 by Sir Joseph Priestly and first synthesized the same year by Sir Humphry Davy. At nitrous oxide parties, Davy, along with such notables as the poets Samuel Coleridge and Robert Southey and the British scholar Peter Roget (author of *Roget's Thesaurus*), experienced the light-headed euphoria and uncontrollable

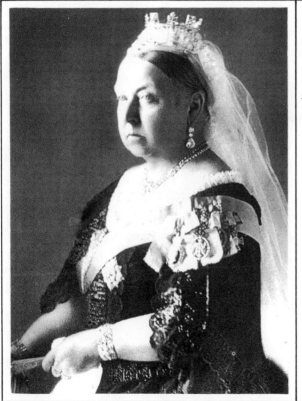

Queen Victoria (1819–1901) conferred the order of knighthood upon Dr. James Simpson after he successfully used chloroform to deaden her pain during his delivery of her eighth child.

fits of laughter that resulted from inhaling the drug—the reason it is often called laughing gas. After one of these parties Southey commented that the highest heaven was certainly saturated with nitrous oxide. In 1799 Davy, observing the drug's pain-reducing property, suggested that it be used during surgery. However, it would be another 45 years before testing for this purpose began.

There are reports of American students using nitrous oxide for recreational purposes in the early 19th century. One student, recognizing its commercial potential, actually quit medical school and went into the nitrous oxide business. He would hold demonstrations and sell the inhalant for 25 cents per dose. At one of these gatherings, Horace Wells, after seeing an intoxicated man seriously injure himself without feeling any pain, realized the drug's potential as an anesthetic. The next day, Wells inhaled some nitrous oxide and felt no

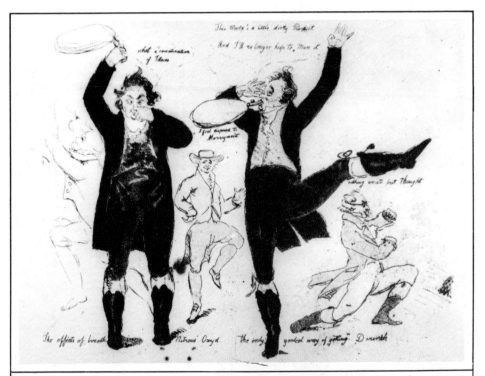

An early 19th-century cartoon depicting the ridiculous behavior of men under the influence of nitrous oxide. Not so funny, however, were the many headlines of the 1960s reporting deaths due to inhalant abuse.

discomfort when the student entrepreneur pulled one of his teeth—an experience Wells realized would forever change dentistry.

Ether

Ether was often prescribed as a medicinal agent in the later 1800s. Interestingly, it was often consumed as a liquid, and early accounts described "ether frolics" during which groups of people would drink ether as if it were a liqueur.

One such report is of a woman whose doctor prescribed ether in the form of a syrup to relieve menstrual complications. She took it often during a 4-month period, but then abstained from using it for 20 years. When ether was again prescribed to alleviate anemia and gastric pains, the woman became accustomed to keeping a small bottle with her at all times, from which she could inhale whenever the pain became unbearable. During a 4-year period, her doses quickly increased until she was chronically intoxicated. Her character changed dramatically, and she began to lead a life of solitude and idleness. When not under the influence of the ether, she would fall into a state of depression. However, as soon as she inhaled more of the drug, she would quickly become gay and talkative. Finally, the police found her on the streets of Paris begging for money to satisfy her 4-year-old ether habit. In a state of complete mental and physical degeneration, she was

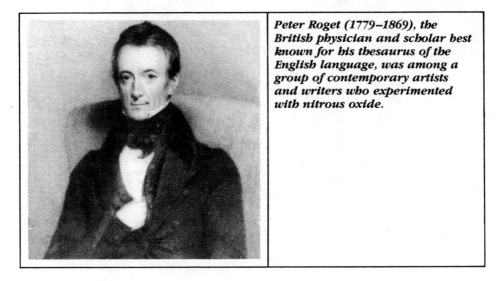

Peter Roget (1779–1869), the British physician and scholar best known for his thesaurus of the English language, was among a group of contemporary artists and writers who experimented with nitrous oxide.

admitted to a clinic. Total abstinence resulted in full recovery, and when she was released a few months later, she had lost her craving for ether.

Other Painkillers and Solvents

Many incidents of solvent abuse were reported between the mid-1800s and the mid-1900s. In most of these cases, excessive, compulsive drug use grew out of legitimate treatment for a medical problem. In one example, a doctor prescribed *trichloroethylene*, a painkiller and anesthetic, to treat a man's facial twitch. After several days of repeated use, the man began taking the drug for its mind-altering effects. Another case involved a man who inhaled chloroform to relieve headaches resulting from a brain concussion. Although he claimed to be taking the drug only to relieve his pain, his habit developed into the daily use of 100 grams. On at least one occasion, he consumed an entire bottle and remained unconscious for four days.

While the use of volatile organic solvents was well known by the beginning of the 20th century, the compulsive

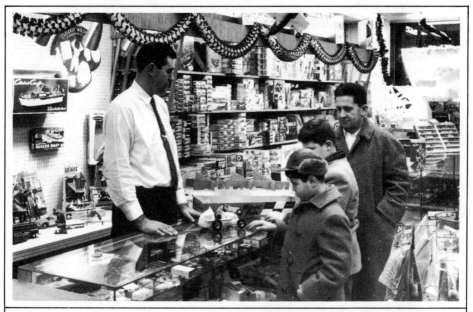

Toy shops and stationery stores often carry airplane glue and typewriter correction fluid, products that can cause sickness, delirium, and even death when used for their intoxicating effects.

nature of this practice was not yet recognized as a form of drug abuse. Solvent abuse by large populations was not reported in scientific literature until the early 1950s. Although many claim that solvent, and especially propellant (see below), abuse in the United States started in California, in fact, the earliest accounts came from the East Coast. One such account describes an outbreak of gasoline sniffing in Warren, Pennsylvania, in the late 1940s. During the 1950s and 1960s an increasing number of articles appeared in newspapers and magazines describing adolescents sniffing airplane glue. Toluene, the active, mind-altering solvent in glue, was subsequently removed from glue and many spray paints.

Popular Inhalants Today

In 1962 the first case of glue sniffing in Great Britain was reported. A 20-year-old man started inhaling glue and after 18 months had increased his dose from one-third of a tube per week to 2 tubes per night. This high dosage produced hallucinations. When he tried to stop using the drug he experienced the DTs, or *delirium tremens*, a violent form of drug withdrawal often experienced by alcoholics and characterized by confusion, restlessness, sweating, tremors, and hallucinations. After sniffing 6 tubes, the man became semicomatose and was admitted to a clinic, where he recovered. However, soon after being released he resumed the habit.

Various aerosols, gases, propellants, and refrigerants also found their way into the solvent-abuser repertoire. These inhalants became popular because they could be found in common household items in which they were used to pressurize soft foods, such as canned whipped cream. Some of these inhalants have the interesting side effect of changing the pitch of the user's voice. At first, many of these propellants were considered to be inert, or to have no effect on the body, and thus their effects were thought to be caused by anoxia. However, the intoxication produced by these inhalants resembles that produced by alcohol, a fact that supports the belief that these substances do indeed affect bodily systems.

Aerosols and propellants continued to rise in popularity. Eventually, it seemed that almost every type of aerosol was being inhaled, including glass chillers, vegetable nonstick frying pan sprays, cold-weather engine starters, air sanitizers, window cleaners, furniture polishes, insecticides, disinfectants, spray medications, deodorants, hair sprays, and antiperspirants.

One of the most continuously popular inhalants has been the gas nitrous oxide. When inhaled in small amounts, this substance produces a light-headed, drifting feeling which lasts but for a few seconds. During the 1960s and 1970s a popular party activity was to fill plastic garbage bags with the gas and pass them from person to person. A few deep breaths provided an exhilarating "rush." Nitrous oxide is not obtained as easily as other volatile organic solvents. The increased awareness of this substance's high abuse potential has resulted in tighter restrictions that have further decreased its availability.

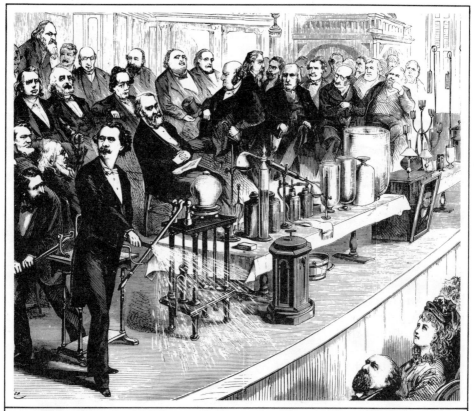

An 1873 etching depicts Horace Wells conducting a public demonstration of the effects of nitrous oxide. Members of the general public were asked to participate by inhaling the laughing gas.

More recently, volatile nitrites, including amyl nitrite (used by heart patients) and butyl nitrite, have become popular in certain circles, particularly among male homosexuals. Though there is little scientific evidence to support abusers' reports of its stimulant effects, it is known that these substances have pronounced cardiovascular and muscle-relaxant effects (see Chapter 5).

By now a long list of abused volatile agents has been created which includes various contact cements and adhesives, paints, lacquers and their thinners, dry cleaning fluids and spot removers, shoe polishes, transmission and brake fluids, liquid waxes and wax removers, degreasers, and refrigerants. Because these types of chemicals are essential to many everyday functions, it remains difficult to control all of them. Perhaps even more alarming is that instead of creating new substances that lack psychoactive, toxic, and abusive properties, each year manufacturers produce many new solvents that have a high abuse potential. This rise in the number of volatile organic solvents increases the likelihood that for certain populations the inhalation form of drug abuse will become even more widespread.

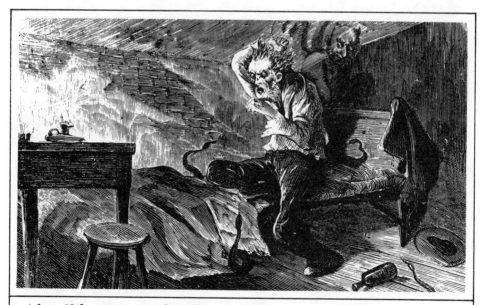

A late 19th-century woodcut illustrates the terrifying symptoms of delirium tremens, or DTs. Some inhalants can produce similar results.

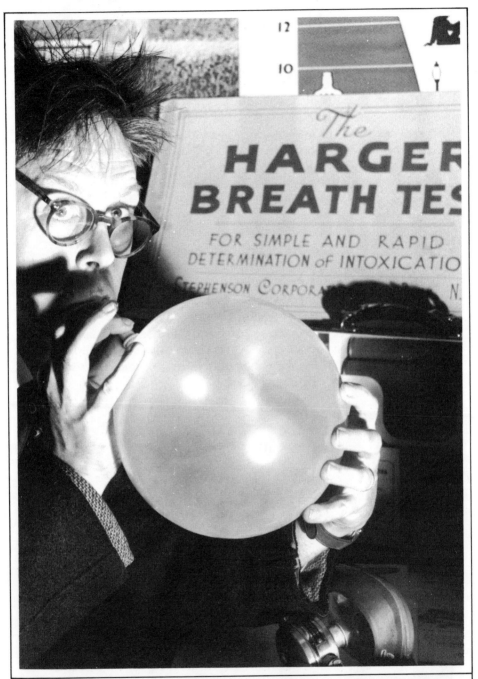

A man blows into a balloon in a demonstration of a breath analyzer. By gauging the color change of a chemical powder encased in a glass tube, the device measures the percentage of alcohol in the body and thus helps determine the degree of intoxication.

CHAPTER 2

THE CHEMISTRY AND PHARMACOLOGY OF SOLVENTS

Volatile organic solvents are usually inhaled and absorbed by the lungs, from where they are transported by the bloodstream to the parts of the body. The process by which solvents produce their mind-altering and/or behavioral effects consists of a fascinating yet complex series of events influenced by such factors as the type of exposure; the solvent's concentration and chemical properties, which include volatility and solubility; and the body's ability to absorb, distribute, and eliminate the solvent.

Volatility

Volatility is a measure of a substance's tendency to vaporize, or leave the liquid state and enter the gaseous state. A compound with high volatility will vaporize at a relatively low temperature, such as at room temperature. When a highly volatile liquid is placed in a closed container, a certain amount of the liquid evaporates, creating a specific pressure, called *vapor pressure*, within the container. The greater the vapor pressure, the more readily a substance will enter the gaseous state. For example, ether, which has a high vapor pressure and is a liquid at room temperature, will evaporate rapidly if it is left in an open dish. When a liquid enters the gaseous state, it is usually measured in parts per million (ppm, the number of gas molecules per one million molecules of air; see Table 1).

Table 1

Properties of Solvents of Abuse

COMPOUND CLASS AND NAMES	VAPOR PRESSURE (mm/Hg)	SOLUBILITY (gm/100 ml water)	SATURATION (% in air)	BOILING POINT (°C)	TLV* (ppm)
Aliphatic hydrocarbons					
n-hexane	150	.23	19.7	68.7	500
n-heptane	47.7	.5	6.3	98.4	500
n-octane	10.45	.14	1.4	127.7	500
Aromatic hydrocarbons					
benzene	100	.082	13.15	80.1	25
toluene	30	.047	3.94	110.6	200
o-xylene	10	insoluble	1.32	144.4	200
Halogenated hydrocarbons					
chloroform	200	1.0	na	61.3	50
trichloroethylene	77	.1	10.2	87.0	100
carbon tetrachloride	113	.08	15	76.8	25
Ketones					
acetone	226.3	infinite	29.8	56.1	1000
methyl ethyl ketone	100	25.6	13.2	79.6	200
methyl n-butyl ketone	3.6	1.6	0.5	127.5	100
Alcohols					
methyl alcohol	160	infinite	21.1	64.5	200
ethyl alcohol	50	infinite	6.6	78.4	1000
isopropyl alcohol	44	infinite	5.8	82.4	400
Miscellaneous agents					
freon	gas	5.7	100	−28.0	1000
ether	438.9	6.05	68	34.6	400
amyl nitrate	5	.3	na	150	none

*Threshold Limit Value, or the maximum concentration allowed in the workplace per 8-hour day.

Solubility

Volatile solvents can also be described in terms of the maximum concentration (the saturation point) that can be achieved under a given set of conditions. For example, when air is saturated with water, the humidity is 100%; at this point no more water can evaporate into the air. Some solvents can only achieve a concentration of 1% before saturating the air. Other solvents do not saturate the air until 10% to 30% concentrations are attained. A comparison of the vapor pressures and maximum concentrations of various solvents within subclasses (see Table 1) reveals that these two measures are directly related—a high vapor pressure is associated with a relatively high maximum saturation.

The notion of saturation is important in a discussion of inhalants because the concentration of solvent in the air is directly related to how much the lungs can absorb. For example, the highest concentration of ethanol (ethyl alcohol) that can be attained is about 6.6%. This level is quite irritating, though it can be tolerated for short periods without significant risk to the individual. This is one reason why most people drink, rather than try to inhale, alcohol.

Potency

Solvents also vary in potency. Within the various classes of solvents in Table 1, it appears that the more volatile the substance (and thus the greater the maximum concentration), the less potent it is. The results from early studies suggest that potency is related to the chemical structure of the solvents. As the number of carbon atoms increases so does potency, though after eight carbon atoms, the potency decreases.

In sufficient concentrations, most, but not all, solvents will ignite or explode when exposed to a flame. Because these drugs have the tendency to decrease the user's awareness of this danger, many inhalant abusers have suffered from severe burns. In addition, burns have resulted from the explosion of solvents used in the production of other abused drugs, such as PCP or free-base cocaine (a combination of cocaine and ether). The flammability of volatile anesthetics, such as ether, also makes them very dangerous to use in the operating room. The recent development of nonflammable anesthetics has decreased the risk of fire. Unfortunately, however, some of these nonflammable substances pose other risks, including an increased susceptibility to liver problems.

When a solvent is inhaled, the size of the dose that the body receives depends on its solubility, which is related to certain chemical properties of the inhalant. One important property is the drug's ability to mix with water, blood, or tissue. Many alcohols will mix completely with water. This means that a volume of the alcohol will mix with an equal volume of water. Toluene, however, will only mix at a rate of 0.047 gm (grams) per 100 ml (milliliters) of water, at which point the solution is saturated. On the other hand, alcohol and toluene mix quite well. Table 1 shows the solubility of some volatile organic solvents in water. A comparison between these data and Figure 2 reveals that, in most cases, within solvent classes the greater the size of the molecule, the less soluble it is in water.

The first step in the absorption of the solvent from the air into the body occurs in the lungs (see Figure 1). The concentration of solvent that passes from the lungs to the arterial blood (blood that moves away from the heart in the arteries) is related to the solvent's solubility in blood. As with water, blood solubility is specific to each solvent. For those solvents that are less soluble, the arterial concentration rapidly reaches the inhaled concentration. Solvents that are highly soluble, such as ether, require more time to reach maximum solubility. Thus, in surgical applications first a high concentration of ether is given to reach rapidly the desired level of anesthesia. This is then followed by concentrations just high enough to maintain that level. During solvent sniffing, an abuser inhales very high concentrations, but generally

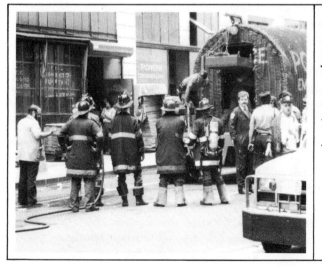

Police, firemen, and members of the bomb squad converge in front of a New York City building, where a barrel of acetone being used in the illegal processing of cocaine exploded in flames, causing considerable damage.

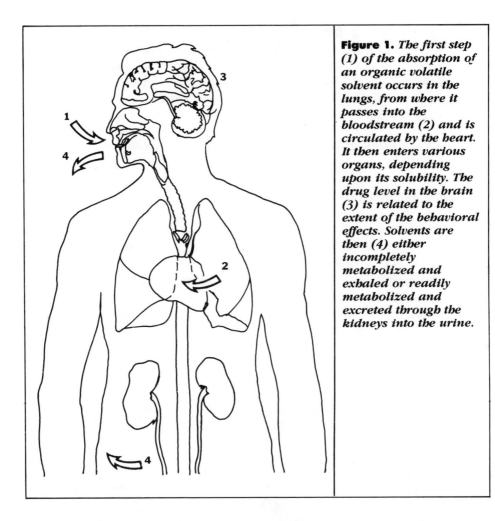

Figure 1. *The first step (1) of the absorption of an organic volatile solvent occurs in the lungs, from where it passes into the bloodstream (2) and is circulated by the heart. It then enters various organs, depending upon its solubility. The drug level in the brain (3) is related to the extent of the behavioral effects. Solvents are then (4) either incompletely metabolized and exhaled or readily metabolized and excreted through the kidneys into the urine.*

these doses are separated by intervals long enough to allow the blood/solvent concentration to decrease. This prevents a rapid accumulation of the solvent in the body.

Solubility also affects the solvent's movement from the blood to the parts of the body. Many solvents are highly lipophilic, or chemically attracted to fats. Usually this also means that they are more soluble in fats than in water and will therefore readily leave the blood and accumulate in fatty tissue, such as that of the brain, heart, liver, and muscles. Thus, after the body is exposed to a solvent for a prolonged period of time, significant amounts of solvent will be found in the fat. When exposure is discontinued and solvent/tissue concentrations decline, these stored compounds will slowly leave the fat and produce their effects on the body. For example, nurses and doctors who are exposed to low concentrations of the surgical anesthetic *halothane* during surgery may continue to show levels of the anesthetic for several days after leaving the hospital.

Properties of Solvents

The *pharmacokinetic* properties of solvents determine how these compounds are taken up into the body, distributed, and finally eliminated. Many of the early studies of the pharmacokinetic properties of solvents were done with gaseous anesthetics, such as ether, because of their popularity as surgical aids. Like most volatile organic solvents, anesthetics administered at high doses and for prolonged periods gradually decrease all normal bodily functions, starting with the user's behavior and followed by his or her sensory abilities and reflex functions, such as breathing. Although intentional sol-

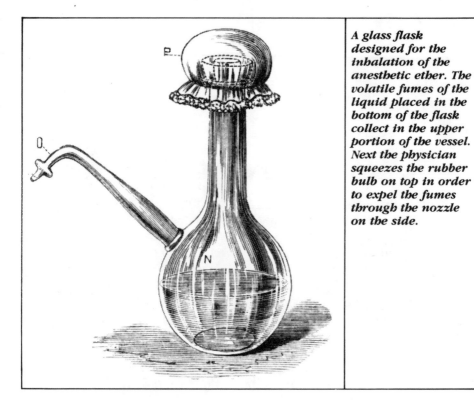

A glass flask designed for the inhalation of the anesthetic ether. The volatile fumes of the liquid placed in the bottom of the flask collect in the upper portion of the vessel. Next the physician squeezes the rubber bulb on top in order to expel the fumes through the nozzle on the side.

vent inhalation might be expected to be terminated by a loss of consciousness, continued inhalation within a confined space might easily result in death. These early studies showed that an accidental overdose could be caused by a dose that was either too high or given too rapidly, and that a safe and effective level of anesthesia could be maintained by regulating the dosage.

A solvent's rate of induction (how quickly the drug takes effect) and rate of recovery (how quickly the effects wear off) depend on the rate of change in its concentration in the brain, all of which directly affect the drug's action on the body. The concentration of volatile organic solvent in the brain is determined by several factors, the most important of which is the concentration of the drug in the arterial blood. This, in turn, is determined by four other factors: the concentration of the solvent in the air; the user's breathing rate; the solubility of the solvent; and the amount of absorption of the drug from arterial blood to body tissues.

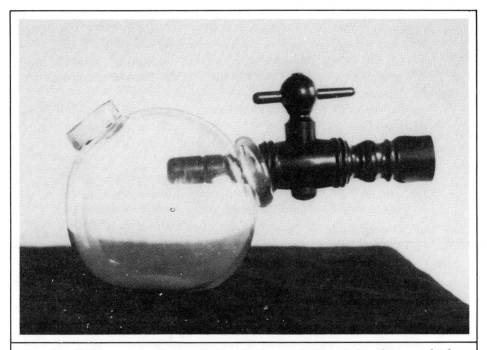

The noted 19th-century dentist William Morton designed this device, which administers a measured amount of ether for anesthetic purposes.

Distribution of Solvents in the Body

Theoretically, when a solvent is inhaled for a sufficient time, its concentration in the air and the body should become equal. However, if the user's rate of breathing or blood flow increases, larger concentrations of solvent in the body will result. Therefore, physical activity or general excitement may increase the effects or the rate of induction of an inhaled drug.

As explained earlier, during solvent inhalation the drug readily passes from the lungs into the blood, which then carries the drug directly to the brain. When a drug is injected or swallowed, it must first pass through the liver, which often detoxifies, or metabolizes, the substance by breaking it up into inactive compounds. Because an inhaled drug moves directly to the brain and therefore is neither diluted nor metabolized, the effects are stronger than those produced by injected or swallowed substances.

Once the drug is in the blood, it is absorbed by the tissues with which it comes into contact. The amount absorbed is determined by the properties of both the drug and tissue. In tissues low in fat content, the solvent concentration will remain approximately equal to its concentration in the blood. But, since most solvents are very lipophilic, solvent concentrations in fat-rich areas such as the brain, liver, and fat deposits will be high.

Another factor in the distribution of solvents is the rate of blood flow in the tissue. Solvents will diffuse more rapidly into tissues with many blood vessels, such as the lungs, brain, heart, and kidneys. Therefore, during exposure to an inhalant the concentration of the drug in these tissues rises rapidly. Because the liver and intestines have fewer blood vessels, solvent concentrations rise much more slowly in them. And finally, solvent concentrations rise even more slowly in muscular and fatty tissues.

The distribution of a solvent can be traced scientifically by labeling it with a radioactive element and following its movement through the body. Not surprisingly, this method has shown that, in addition to solubility and blood flow, distribution depends on the length of exposure. Even though solvents tend to diffuse into more fat-soluble tissues, the rate of flow within these tissues is inversely proportional to the time it takes to get there.

COMMON VOLATILE ORGANIC SOLVENTS

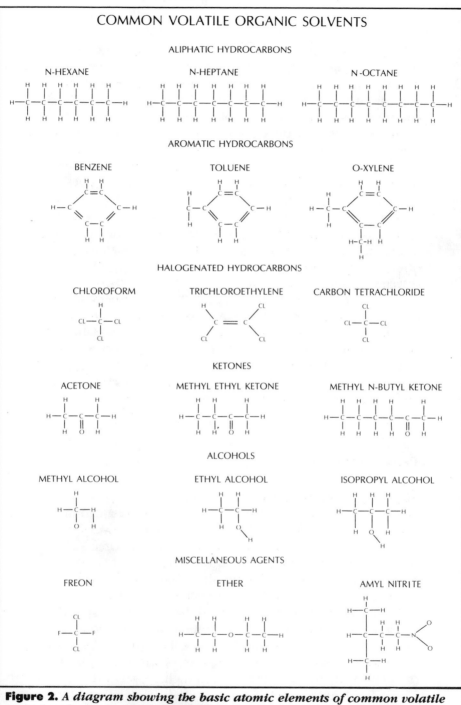

Figure 2. *A diagram showing the basic atomic elements of common volatile organic solvents. Some studies suggest that the potency of each solvent is related to the chemical structure of the molecule.*

Once the solvent is in the body it can leave by different routes (see Figure 1). Many solvents are primarily eliminated by exhaling them, and therefore the factors such as solubility, ventilation rate, and blood flow that influence uptake (absorption) also affect the rate of elimination. As mentioned earlier, solvents seek out those tissues in which they are most soluble. Because these areas are frequently less well supplied by the blood, it takes longer for the solvent to build up there. However, once exposure is terminated the process goes in reverse and stored solvents also leave less readily.

Many solvents are metabolized into a more water-soluble form and excreted as harmless by-products in the urine or passed out of the body through the skin. Unfortunately, some of these by-products are more active and thus more harmful than the original solvent. For example, alcohol is metabolized to *acetaldehyde*, a very toxic agent that is normally eliminated very rapidly from the body. When it is not eliminated, as in those users who have an inherited inability to metabolize ethanol, a drink or two will make the drinker very sick. In fact, a drug called disulfiram (Antabuse), which slows the metabolism of acetaldehyde and thus makes drinking an unpleasant experience, has been used to treat alcohol abuse.

Behavioral Effects

Although scientists understand the process by which many chemical properties of volatile organic solvents relate to their uptake, distribution, and elimination, they know very little about how inhalants produce their behavioral effects. Evidence is growing to suggest that these solvents do have behavioral effects that resemble those of more commonly known drugs. For example, solvents (including alcohol), barbiturates, and minor tranquilizers all share sedative/hypnotic, anti-anxiety, muscle-relaxant, and anticonvulsant actions. Solvents such as ethanol and toluene can enhance the behavioral effects of barbiturates, minor tranquilizers, and methaqualone (a nonbarbiturate sedative/hypnotic such as Quaalude).

It has been shown that *antagonists* (drugs that block the effects of other drugs) that affect benzodiazepines (a group of minor tranquilizers that includes Valium) can also alter some of the effects of volatile organic solvents. This suggests that some of the mechanisms by which solvents produce their effects are similar to those of minor tranquilizers. Many of benzodiazepine's behavioral effects are known to be caused by the actions of these drugs on specific nerve receptors in the brain that respond to a particular inhibitory *neurotransmitter*. (A neurotransmitter is a substance that carries messages between neurons.) Thus, many of the sedative effects of solvents may be related to their effect on this same neurotransmitter system. But very little is known about how they produce their stimulant and anti-anxiety effects.

Solvents may act on many different neurotransmitter systems in the brain. Basically, it is too soon to say that any one effect of a solvent is produced through these mechanisms. This area of research remains essentially unexplored with respect to the solvents' abuse potential, but it appears to hold great promise for the future. Learning about the neurochemical mechanisms by which solvents produce their behavioral effects may also aid in treating high-dose or overdose patients. If solvent antagonists were found, they could be used to reverse the effects of solvent overdose and greatly reduce the chance of an abuser dying or suffering permanent impairment.

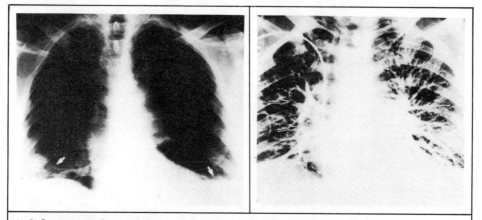

At left is an ordinary chest x-ray. The x-ray on the right was taken after a substance impenetrable to the x-ray was introduced into the patient's bloodstream, allowing a detailed study of the distribution of fluids throughout the body. Using a similar substance, scientists can trace the absorption of inhalants into the body's organs and tissues.

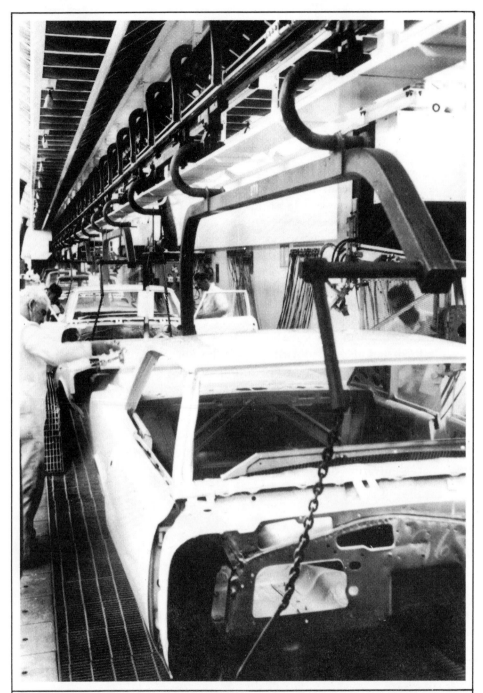

Many factory workers are exposed to a certain amount of solvent fumes on a daily basis. Rotating shifts and the use of face masks lessen the risks of inadvertent solvent inhalation in a factory environment.

CHAPTER 3

EXPOSURE TO THE SOLVENTS

People can come into contact with volatile organic solvents in different ways. With some solvents a single acute, or brief, exposure to relatively high concentrations will produce behavioral effects, whereas prolonged or repeated exposure to substantially lower levels of the same solvent may be more likely to promote cancer or liver disease. This difference suggests that the threshold for producing a particular effect may vary according to the type of exposure and the concentration of solvent in the air.

All solvents do not produce the same effects in the same sequence. For example, one solvent may produce behavioral effects with acute exposures, and adverse health consequences after repeated low-level exposures. Conversely, another solvent may produce adverse health consequences after acute exposures, and behavioral effects only after many low-level exposures. However, one thing is true for all inhalants—repeated exposure to high concentrations will always produce some effect.

Generally, the solvent abuser places a container or rag soaked with the solvent over his or her nose and repeatedly takes short, deep breaths. This pattern, repeated once or twice a minute until the desired behavioral effect is achieved, results in an overall gradual rise in solvent concentration in the body and a rapid rise and fall in solvent concentration in the blood.

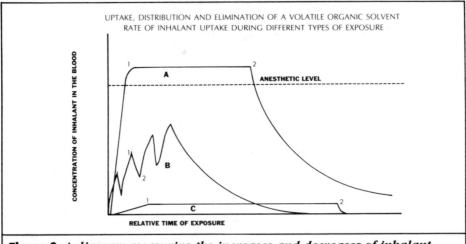

Figure 3. *A diagram measuring the increases and decreases of inhalant levels in the bloodstream over a period of time for three kinds of solvent users: (A) persons being anesthetized, (B) inhalant abusers, and (C) persons who experience exposures on the job.*

This type of exposure differs considerably from the type a person experiences both in certain industrial settings and from an anesthesiologist. In the factory where solvents are legitimately used, concentrations are usually low, yet the duration of exposure may be as great as 8 hours per day. Though this may result in less accumulation of the solvent in the workers' bodies, the solvent's by-products present in the body may produce behavioral changes. An anesthesiologist initially induces anesthesia by administering to the patient a high concentration of the drug, followed by a dose that will maintain a constant level of the anesthetic in the blood.

The abuser inhales solvent concentrations comparable to those administered by the anesthesiologist, but only intermittently (see Figure 3). The abuser's pattern of inhalation allows peak concentrations to occur, but with less danger of accumulation than if he or she were to use it the way the anesthesiologist administers it. With long continuous exposures, both the solvent and its by-products can continue to increase in concentration in the blood and body fat. Prolonged exposure to many of the anesthetics can result in overdosing, causing death if the concentration is kept too high and/or the duration of exposure is too long.

As mentioned earlier, an individual's level of activity during exposure to a solvent can influence how that drug will affect his or her behavior. Both an increase in lung intake, which brings more solvent in contact with the blood, and an increase in blood flow contribute to higher drug levels in the body. For example, recent studies have shown that the amount of solvent in the blood can be nearly doubled by riding a bicycle during exposure. The effects of solvents can also be increased by holding one's breath, which raises the amount of carbon dioxide in the blood, increases the relative amount of solvent in the blood, and also produces a small amount of anoxia.

Inhalation is not the only means by which a volatile organic solvent can be ingested. Some studies have measured the effects of injecting solvents into the body, applying them directly to the skin, or drinking them. Though the effects are frequently very similar to those produced by inhalation, some differences have been observed. For example, though applying toluene to the skin will produce this drug's characteristic effects, it also causes skin irritation so painful that the user will probably not repeat the experience.

The method of administration will also determine how quickly the solvent gets into the bloodstream and how rapidly it is broken down into its by-products. With routes of administration other than inhalation, the skin and/or the gastrointestinal system are involved, both of which absorb inhalants relatively slowly. On the other hand, these substances readily

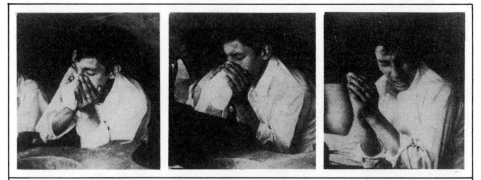

A teenager sniffing glue. Fumes from the toluene in the glue can irritate the mucous membranes around the eyes and nose. Repeated exposure leads to tissue ulceration and respiratory problems.

pass from the lungs into the bloodstream during inhalation. Since the speed at which a drug produces its effects is directly related to its abuse potential, inhalation remains the most popular route of administration among solvent abusers.

The Effects of Repeated Exposures

Situational variables are also important in determining the effects of a drug. If a person repeatedly uses inhalants, not only will the drug accumulate in the body, but the solvent may become associated with a certain place, person, or thing present during exposure to the drug. When this occurs, the presence of one or more of these environmental factors may uniquely influence the solvent's effects. For example, in a familiar environment a heroin addict will be able to tolerate a certain dose, above which the effects become dangerous or even lethal. However, in a completely novel environment this same dose may kill the addict.

The most typical effect of repeated exposure is the development of *tolerance*. Tolerance is defined as a decrease in susceptibility to the effects of a drug due to its continual

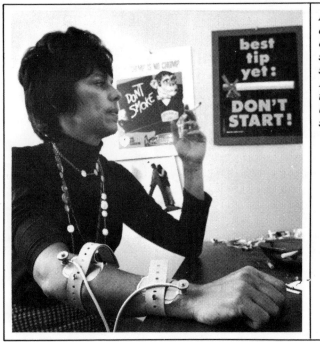

A woman attempts to quit smoking by enduring an electric shock every time she takes a puff. A conditioned aversion to inhalants can also be attained by using such extreme methods.

administration, resulting in the user's need to increase the drug dosage in order to achieve the effects experienced previously. There are two types of tolerance: physiological and behavioral. With physiological tolerance the body adapts to the presence of a drug, either by producing more enzymes to metabolize, or break down, the drug more quickly or by producing more nerve receptors to offset the drug's effects.

Though many drugs produce both physiological and behavioral tolerance, there is little evidence that inhalant use leads to either type of tolerance. One exception, however, is alcohol, for which both types occur. Further research is needed to explore the distinction between alcohol and the other inhalants and the possibility that tolerance does exist.

Repeated solvent exposures can also produce *sensitivity*, whereby relatively low concentrations of the drug are able to produce effects similar to the ones initially produced only by higher concentrations.

Conditioned Aversion

Repeated exposure to a solvent can also result in the emergence of its noxious properties. Many drugs have aversive properties (effects that make a user avoid using the drug) that seem related to their ability to make people sick. When one of these drugs is first used and causes illness or an unpleasant experience, a person may develop a reluctance to approach specific aspects of the environment in which the drug was first ingested. Clinically, this phenomenon is known as *conditioned aversion*. This phenomenon has been well demonstrated in people taking very noxious agents such as anti-cancer drugs. In one series of studies, children suffering from cancer were offered their choice of several flavors of ice cream just before undergoing chemotherapy, a type of treatment that can cause great discomfort. When several months later the same children were again offered ice cream, they rejected those flavors they had initially chosen. Studies using animals have demonstrated that conditioned aversion learning can be a way to change behavior.

Unfortunately, there are few examples of conditioned aversions resulting from the inhalation of volatile organic solvents (see Chapter 4). However, this may be because relatively few researchers have studied the behavioral effects of these substances.

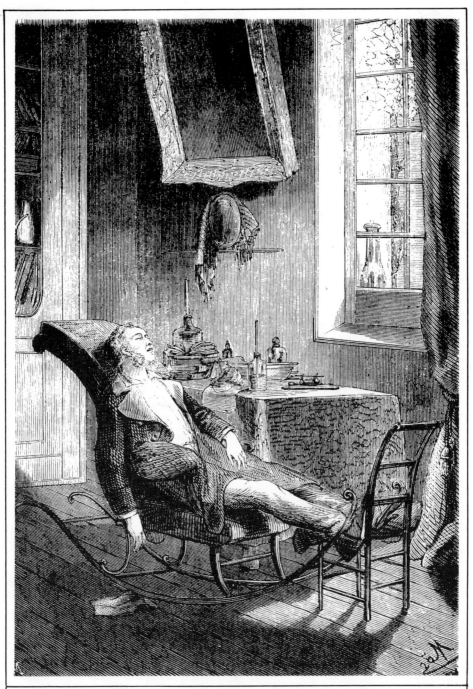

A 19th-century etching depicts a French scientist who has fallen fast asleep in his drawing room after inhaling ether in an experiment to determine the anesthetic effects of the solvent.

CHAPTER 4

THE BEHAVIORAL EFFECTS OF INHALANTS

Behavior is often controlled by various aspects of the environment. This seemingly obvious fact has made it possible for scientists to develop a science of behavior called *behavioral psychology*. Psychologists in this field are able to identify different behaviors, characterize how they are controlled, and determine how a change in the environment affects a normally occurring behavior. In the mid-1950s the field of behavioral psychology expanded to include behavioral pharmacology, the study of the effects of drugs on behavior. Because of the technological advances in science, researchers were at last able to finely control behavior and detect even very small drug effects. With these new capabilities they could measure the role of behavior in producing these drug effects.

Two of the more interesting pharmacological discoveries are that (1) the effects of a drug may depend more on *how* the behavior is controlled than *why* the behavior occurs and (2) some drugs will affect certain behaviors in a particular way while other drugs will not. With this information, scientists are able to identify different types of drugs on the basis of how they affect behavior as well as develop new drugs that have specific behavioral effects.

One area of behavioral pharmacology is the study of the behavioral consequences of drugs. Researchers have found that animals will work for food and/or drugs, just as people will. In fact, many of the drugs abused by people can be used to reinforce an animal's behavior or support their drug-seeking behavior.

Direct and Indirect Behavioral Effects

The behavioral effects produced by drugs can be either direct or indirect. A drug's direct effects are those that immediately alter the user's physical or psychological state. If the individual desires to use the drug again, the substance is said to produce *drug-seeking* or *drug-reinforced* behaviors. Conversely, a drug can produce *drug-avoiding* behaviors, in which case an individual does not seek, and often actively avoids, the drug. A drug's indirect effects influence other, usually non-drug related, behaviors, such as those associated with school or work.

Drugs, including inhalants, can either increase or decrease these behaviors. However, these effects may only be obtained over a limited range of doses or concentrations. Thus, a drug may have no effect below a certain level, may produce obvious effects when the dose rises above another level, and may suppress certain behavior at even higher doses. Not only are researchers able to relate a drug's direct and indirect effects to the dose, but they can relate a drug's behavioral effects with its other toxic effects. The branch of

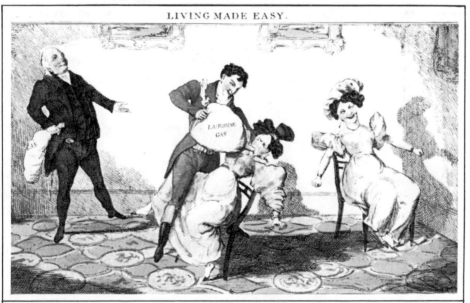

LIVING MADE EASY.

A rather chauvinistic cartoon provides a humorous look at the feeling of euphoria produced by the inhalation of laughing gas.

behavioral pharmacology that studies the adverse consequences of exposure to toxins is called *toxicology*.

Using animals in experiments to determine the effects of drugs allows researchers to gain a greater understanding of inhalants without exposing people to potential dangers. In addition, though in humans it is impossible to control behavioral and drug histories, as well as genetic, environmental, and dietary factors, they can be controlled in research that uses animal subjects. Because of the emergence of better techniques in animal studies, behavioral pharmacology and behavioral toxicology are beginning to produce a great deal of useful and dependable information related to the direct and indirect effects of solvents.

Applying inhalant self-administration procedures to animals requires tremendous technical skills as well as a good deal of knowledge of the solvents themselves. To be able to apply the data collected from animal studies to humans, the

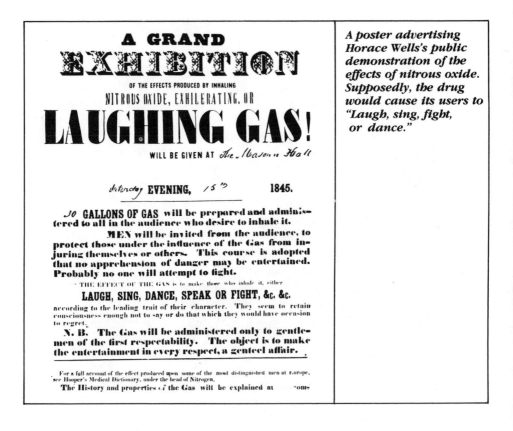

A poster advertising Horace Wells's public demonstration of the effects of nitrous oxide. Supposedly, the drug would cause its users to "Laugh, sing, fight, or dance."

animal's behavior must closely approximate human behavior. Though this is relatively easy if the drug is injected, inhalation poses many problems. Specific concentrations of the inhalant must be delivered accurately and rapidly soon after the animal exhibits drug-seeking behavior. In addition, the level of solvent has to be monitored in order to establish a concentration great enough to reinforce this behavior.

Recent studies show that access to solvents can support self-administration behavior. In one study, monkeys in a closed chamber were trained to press a lever in order to receive a 15-second delivery of toluene. The small size of the chamber made it possible for scientists to measure the concentration of the drug. When the solvent was withheld the lever-pushing behavior disappeared. The monkeys' behavior in many ways mimics the way people would learn to seek a solvent. Similar techniques with monkeys have shown that nitrous oxide can also support self-administration. Such studies demonstrate that the study of self-administration of solvents is practical, and yet there have been few studies of the reinforcing properties of other volatile organic solvents.

Inhalants can have direct noxious effects, and these can affect the user in one of two ways. First, use of a particular solvent can cause a person or animal to avoid further contact with that drug. In this case, the solvent is serving as a negative reinforcer, such that behavior that terminates solvent delivery is reinforced. Experiments have shown that, when given the opportunity, mice will turn off the delivery of formaldehyde, thereby demonstrating that this substance's noxious properties reinforce behavior that terminates contact with the drug. Similar scientific methods could be used to determine at which levels solvents may be irritating or aversive.

Alternatively, if exposure to a solvent is a consequence of a specific behavior, subsequent contact with this solvent will decrease that behavior. In this case, the drug is functioning as a punisher. Scolding and spanking are common punishers, though they are only true punishers if they decrease the behavior for which the child is being disciplined. The examples of conditioned aversions in the previous chapter are similar to punishment—when a neutral taste or smell is paired with a noxious event, the taste or smell becomes a conditioned punisher. Several volatile organic solvents have been shown to have these types of noxious properties. For example, when the delivery of several halogenated hydro-carbons, such as trichloroethylene, is paired with a distinctive taste, foods with that taste are subsequently avoided. Very little is known about how various substances produce con-ditioned aversions, but this response clearly demonstrates their noxious properties.

Interestingly, many drugs have both reinforcing and pun-ishing properties. For example, in one experiment, 60% to 80% nitrous oxide was used to establish a conditioned aver-sion, while in another experiment 30% to 75% nitrous oxide had reinforcing properties. Thus, it appears that 60% to 75% of this drug can be either punishing or reinforcing. In studies using other drugs, similar concentrations have been shown to serve as reinforcers and punishers in the same animal. It has also been demonstrated that environmentally relevant stimuli, such as food or electric shock, can also function in this apparently paradoxical fashion. Therefore, it cannot be assumed that a drug will have reinforcing or punishing effects independent of the conditions under which it is administered.

In the past, the noxious effect of a drug was thought to be related to its natural ability to produce sickness in the

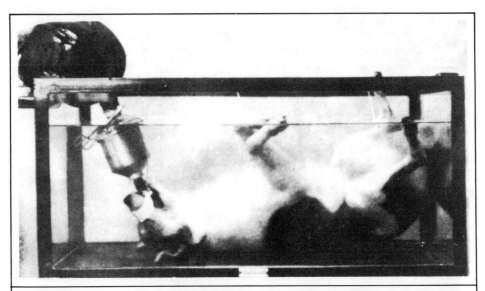

An anesthetized dog, connected to a breathing apparatus, sleeps peacefully under water. Experiments involving animals and inhalants have advanced the study of these drugs' effects upon humans.

user. Although this aversive effect does often appear during initial exposures to inhalants, it is very interesting that some individuals become ill but go on to become solvent abusers, while others become ill and never again sniff an inhalant. Many psychologists think that initial experiences with some drugs can strongly predispose some individuals to either take or not take those drugs again. Behavioral experiments have emphasized that prior experience can be a strong determinant in establishing conditioned aversions. For individuals with prior experience with either the drug or the taste stimulus paired with drug delivery, larger doses are required to produce conditioned aversion, if it can be produced at all.

Some individuals may react differently than other individuals to certain drugs. It is well established that some individuals cannot tolerate alcohol or other drugs to the extent that others can. While this distinction has traditionally been regarded as being caused by a possible difference in the genetic makeup of these people, it may also be a result of their prior experience with drugs. In addition, if different drugs can produce similar effects, the prior exposure to one may

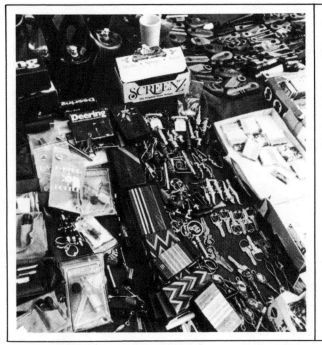

Paraphernalia used in the abuse of several different kinds of drugs on display in the showcase of a contemporary "head shop." Though legal, these stores worsen the widespread problem of drug abuse by making drug-related equipment easily accessible.

increase or decrease the possibility of trying another. This is supported by the fact that most drug users are polydrug users (users of many drugs).

Although solvents can be reinforcing or punishing, little is known about their other direct effects. For example, solvents can also serve as *discriminative stimuli*. This means that in the presence of the smell of a solvent or while experiencing or even observing some behavioral or pharmacological effect of a solvent, a person may be more likely to engage in certain behaviors. For example, solvents may set the occasion for certain social behaviors that are quite different than those that would be seen at home.

Some volatile organic solvents have been assessed for their discriminative properties, and they appear to be similar to those of ethanol and pentobarbital, a short-acting barbiturate. This supports the growing evidence that some of the behavioral effects of solvents are very similar to those of sedative/hypnotic drugs. Future studies that measure the discriminative properties of inhalants may help us better understand the subjective effects of these substances.

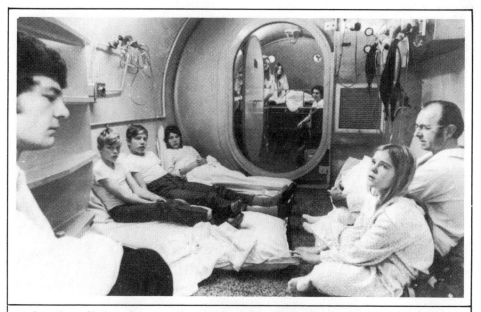

A family suffering from carbon monoxide poisoning due to a leaky furnace pipe in their home recovers in an oxygen room of a hospital.

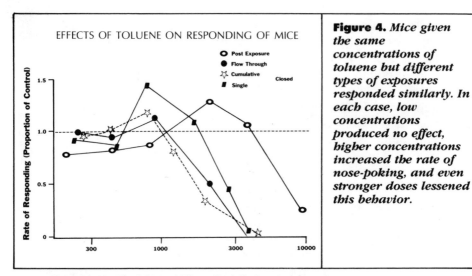

Figure 4. *Mice given the same concentrations of toluene but different types of exposures responded similarly. In each case, low concentrations produced no effect, higher concentrations increased the rate of nose-poking, and even stronger doses lessened this behavior.*

SOURCE: Glowa, John R. "The Behavioral Effects of Volatile Organic Solvents."

Another direct behavioral effect of solvents is that they may produce salivation, tearing, or even nausea. These responses are automatic and clearly indicate the irritating properties of these substances.

Most of the solvents' direct effects are related in some way to their abuse potential. Some scientists have suggested that if an individual's pre-exposure to solvents were carefully controlled it might be possible to play these direct effects off each other. The prior establishment of a solvent's punishing effects may severely disrupt the development of the drug's reinforcing properties, which develop gradually, and thus greatly decrease the incidence of solvent abuse.

Indirect behavioral effects are usually measured by comparing the behavior exhibited while under the influence of a drug with normal behavior, considered to be the behavioral baseline. This baseline is usually characterized in terms of the rate of behavior (the number of responses per unit of time) and the pattern of behavior, both of which can be controlled in an experimental situation. Frequently, the baseline data is made into a graph similar to the one in Figure 4. For example, a hungry mouse will quickly learn to poke its nose into a hole in order to get milk, and the animal's mastering of this task is indicated by an increase in nose-poking. Over time, the rate and pattern of the mouse's behavior will

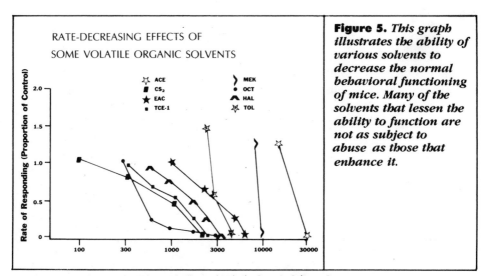

Figure 5. *This graph illustrates the ability of various solvents to decrease the normal behavioral functioning of mice. Many of the solvents that lessen the ability to function are not as subject to abuse as those that enhance it.*

SOURCE: Glowa, John R. "The Behavioral Effects of Volatile Organic Solvents."

stabilize and represent the behavioral baseline. After this has been established, the effects of a solvent on nose-poking behavior can be determined by exposing the mouse to a specific concentration of the drug and comparing the new rate and pattern of behavior to the baseline.

If the experimental subject is exposed to a range of solvent concentrations, the resultant data, when graphed, will produce what is called a concentration-effect curve. This illustrates the range of concentrations over which behavioral effects will occur. Typically solvents will either increase or decrease behavior, depending upon the concentration. One experiment measured the effects of four different types of toluene exposure on mice (see Figure 4). In the first case, the animal was in a closed chamber in which the concentration of toluene was gradually increased. In the second case, the animal was exposed to constant concentrations. In the third, the mouse was in a chamber in which the inhalant was allowed to flow through. And in the last case, the subject was exposed to different concentrations of toluene after having ingested the same solvent shortly before. All four methods of exposure produced similar results. Very low concentrations were found to have no effect, somewhat higher concentrations increased the rate of nose-poking, and still higher toluene concentrations decreased this behavior. For all subjects there existed a certain high dosage which when reached entirely eliminated the nose-poking behavior. Clearly, when it comes to the effects of inhalants on behavior, the type of exposure is less important than the concentration of the drug.

Though some solvents have rate-increasing effects, at relatively high concentrations all solvents can decrease behavior and produce a state that resembles intoxication or anesthesia. This ability to impair normal behavioral functioning is an important effect of solvent exposure because these effects are potentially harmful to anyone exposed to these solvents and engaged in dangerous tasks, such as driving a

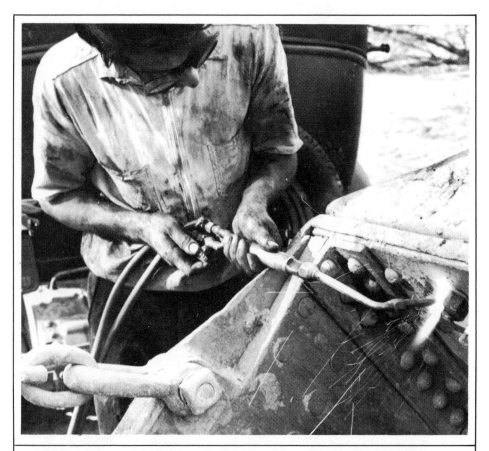

Narcylene is a purified form of acetylene, a gas used in blowtorches. Although it can also serve as an anesthetic, in higher doses narcylene can cause auditory hallucinations.

car or operating machinery. Thus, it is important to determine the concentrations at which the solvents decrease behavior so that safe limits can be set for levels of solvents at the workplace.

Figure 5 illustrates the ability of various solvents to decrease the normal behavioral functioning of mice working for food. One interesting observation is that solvents, such as carbon disulfide, that decrease behavior at lower concentrations are not typically abused. Therefore, it seems that the rate-decreasing effects of solvents are not necessarily related to their abuse potential.

Many of the substances mentioned in Figure 5 will also produce excitatory effects. In fact, current data does support the notion that, as long as the inhalant abuser can limit solvent intake to concentrations that cause rate-increasing effects, it is these effects that most greatly contribute to a solvent's abuse potential.

Subjective Effects in Humans

Because of ethical restraints, there have been few experiments focusing on the effects of solvents on humans. However, there are several anecdotal reports of individuals who sought clinical help for solvent abuse problems. One unusual account is that of a 28-year-old doctor who was experimenting with the anesthetic *narcylene*, a purified form of acetylene. When he ingested the drug the first time, he became intoxicated. His second exposure to the drug produced hallucinations. His investigation continued, but by this time it was no longer just for the purpose of furthering science. The doctor became accustomed to inhaling narcylene solely for the pleasurable state that it induced. In addition to experiencing behavioral changes, he reported frequent auditory hallucinations. After about a month, he began to hallucinate even without the drug, sometimes for as long as five days. It was at this time that he sought medical assistance, and apparently he recovered without any ill effects.

According to this and other clinical case reports, inhalants produce euphoria, or a carefree feeling that removes the user from his or her everyday worries. Users also experience hallucinations, memory loss, and other unpleasant side effects. Sometimes they display aggressiveness. The range of possible effects is large, and even well-controlled studies have not been able to determine if this is due to differences between individual users or if each user may experience different effects on various occasions. In addition, it is not known if during these studies the human subjects were using other drugs that might have altered the inhalants' effects.

Little is known about how inhalants produce their effects. It does not appear that tolerance to these subjective effects occurs. In fact, with repeated exposure they may be intensified and inappropriate behaviors characteristic of psychotic individuals can develop.

In one case, a young pharmacist, who was using chloroform to treat a facial twitch, quickly developed the habit of inhaling the drug to obtain its behavioral effects. Eventually, he was intoxicated almost continuously, and after one

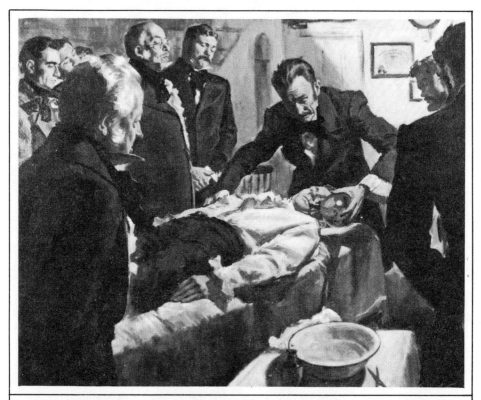

A mid-19th-century painting depicts William Morton using a flask he designed to administer ether to a patient prior to surgery.

13-day binge he began to experience hallucinations, appetite loss, and restlessness. When he vomited blood, the pharmacist reported his case to a clinic. During withdrawal from the drug he became terribly anxious, incoherent, and paranoid, though these symptoms eventually disappeared. When he had fully recovered and left the clinic, he discovered that he had developed a profound aversion to the smell of chloroform.

The inhalants' other subjective effects resemble the sedative effects of barbiturates. When ingested, both barbiturates and opiates produce a dreamy state that makes the individual indifferent to his or her surroundings. This, in turn, allows the individual to escape temporarily the problems in the real world. In fact, this effect may form the basis for initial solvent use. But the use of inhalants or any other drug of abuse will not make the problems disappear. A person must learn to face and seek to change his or her environment, for when the drugs' effects wear off, the problems may appear even more insurmountable.

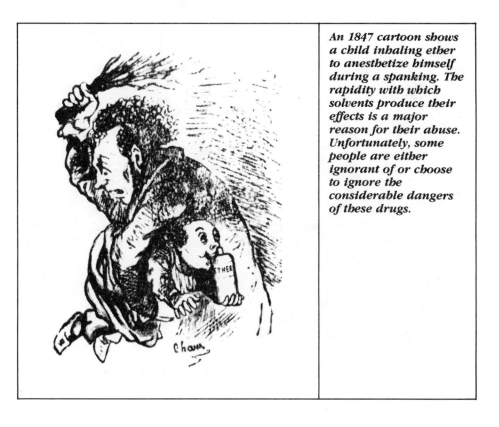

An 1847 cartoon shows a child inhaling ether to anesthetize himself during a spanking. The rapidity with which solvents produce their effects is a major reason for their abuse. Unfortunately, some people are either ignorant of or choose to ignore the considerable dangers of these drugs.

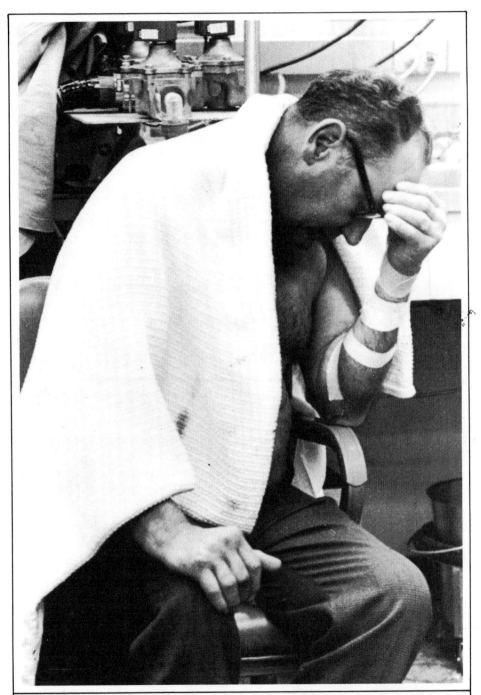

A coal miner who is suffering from black lung disease, an illness caused by the inhalation of coal dust. Similarly, solvent inhalation can destroy cell tissue and disrupt normal functioning of the lungs.

CHAPTER 5

THE HEALTH EFFECTS OF SOLVENT ABUSE

*I*n addition to producing effects that the drug abuser considers to be positive, volatile organic solvents can also produce toxic, or poisonous, effects. It is for this reason that inhalants are also called *toxicants*. These substances can be lethal to individuals who are exposed to them in sufficient concentrations or for long enough durations. Somewhat lower levels can be damaging to major organ systems of the body. Though the desired behavioral effects of some solvents can be obtained at levels below those that may produce dangerous side effects, other solvents have toxic effects at levels below those that produce the desired behavioral effects.

Because many abused solvents contain small quantities of other agents that affect the body, people who use inhalants can never be certain of what risks they are taking. For example, while toluene is toxic to the nervous system only at very high concentrations, at lower levels the benzene that is commonly found with toluene can cause cancer. Therefore, in order to obtain the desired behavioral effects of toluene, the user is exposing him- or herself to toxic levels of benzene.

Teratological Effects

Volatile organic solvents have been shown to have *terato-logical* effects, or adverse effects on the growing fetus, such as physical malformations or functional impairment. Exposure to some inhalants may, in fact, decrease body weight and size and even IQ. Some solvents can be *embryotoxic*, or capable of terminating a pregnancy. And still other solvents can damage reproductive cells and thus prevent conception and pregnancy. In fact, many inhalants can produce all of the effects over a wide range of concentrations. For example, inhaling carbon tetrachloride can result in the death of the fetus or the embryo or, with high doses, even the death of the mother. Sub-lethal doses of benzene have been shown to cause cleft palates in mice.

Only a few inhalants have been systematically tested for their ability to cause prenatal abnormalities or postnatal abnormalities following prenatal exposure. Currently, researchers are studying the learning ability of animals that have been

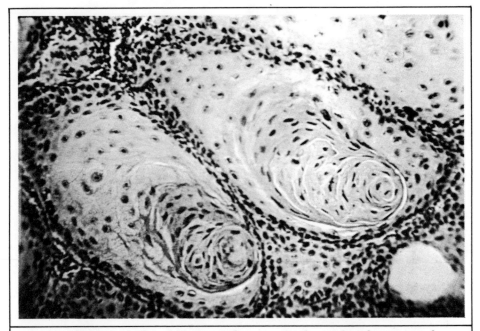

A microphotograph shows an area of cancer in the midst of a group of normal cells. Research on the effects of solvent exposure has suggested that some inhalants are carcinogenic, or cancer causing.

exposed to solvents before birth. Thus far the data suggest that prenatal exposure does affect learning, sometimes dramatically. Clearly, a pregnant woman who inhales volatile organic solvents, either recreationally or at home or at her workplace, is greatly risking her own and her child's life.

Carcinogenic Effects

Recently, there has been growing concern about exposure to solvents because several of them are suspected of being *carcinogens*, or substances that produce or contribute to the growth of cancer. For compounds that can be shown to produce these effects, occupational exposure standards must be

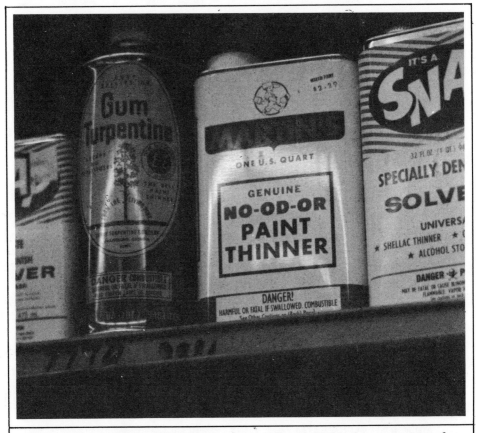

Solvents and thinners that are commercially available for a variety of purposes are often hazardous, and sometimes fatal, when inhaled.

lowered to reduce the potential risk of cancer. Thus far, benzene is the only solvent for which these effects have been extensively studied. Because several other inhalants, including chloroform and formaldehyde, may be carcinogenic, efforts to evaluate all solvents must be intensified.

Cardiovascular Effects

After the initial reports of propellant abuse, follow-up reports from hospitals indicated that inhalation of some volatile organic solvents could result in a syndrome known as *sudden death*. From cases of abusers dying even before reaching the emergency room, researchers discovered that inhalants can have detrimental effects on the normal functioning of the heart.

A number of solvents have been shown to produce *ventricular fibrillation*, an abnormal pumping action of the heart. In dogs, heptane and other inhalants, especially propellants, have been shown to produce *arrhythmia*, or irregular heartbeats. There are several ways in which solvents can interfere with the normal functioning of the heart.

First, the heart can be sensitized to *norepinephrine*, a substance produced in the adrenal glands that is normally released during stressful situations, so that the combination of inhalant use and stress overstimulates the heart. Animal studies that focused on the effect of ether on stress have shown that exposure to this inhalant does in fact lead to a release of norepinephrine and to elevated heart rate and blood pressure.

Second, inhalants, such as the chlorinate hydrocarbons, may depress the ability of the heart muscle to contract. As a result, the body, including the heart, is not supplied with the usual amount of blood.

Finally, the adverse effect on the cardiovascular system may be due to an increase in heart rate, which is caused by irritating the inner lining of the lungs.

Interestingly, some volatile organic solvents can be used to treat cardiovascular difficulties. For example, amyl nitrite is often used to reduce the pain caused by a reduced blood flow to the heart. Though some solvents may be beneficial when used in doses prescribed by a doctor, their abuse can have very serious consequences.

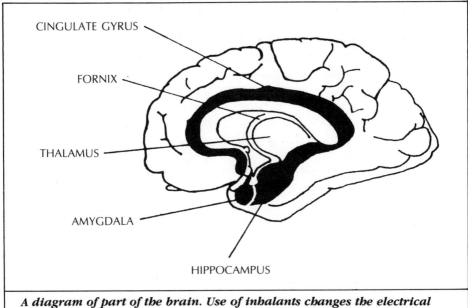

CINGULATE GYRUS

FORNIX

THALAMUS

AMYGDALA

HIPPOCAMPUS

A diagram of part of the brain. Use of inhalants changes the electrical activity within the brain, possibly resulting in hallucinations and convulsions. In addition, the amygdala, the center of emotional behavior, is adversely affected during and after exposure to inhalants.

Effects on Electrical Activity in the Brain

Normal functioning of the brain can be characterized by low levels of electrical activity generated by the continuous firing of neurons, or nerve cells. This activity is readily monitored by placing electrodes on the scalp and amplifying the signals, a technique called *electroencephalography*, or EEG. During the day the overall activity of the brain remains somewhat moderate. If something startling occurs, the electrical activity becomes irregular, characterized by spikes, or sharp pulses, when seen on the graph. During sleep, brain activity decreases, though when there is dreaming this activity may actually be as high as it is during highly excited waking states.

Changes in normally occurring electrical activity in the brain have been related to several neurological abnormalities, some of which are similar to epilepsy. Other changes have been associated with a person's ability to orient him- or herself and concentrate. In laboratory studies, exposure to solvents causes a change in EEG activity in two areas of the brain: the frontal cortex, where sensory information is processed, and the reticular formation, the area associated with arousal levels. Repeated exposure to inhalants has especially pronounced effects on electrical activity in the reticular formation. In addition, the *amygdala*, an area in the brain associated with emotional behavior, is affected during and after repeated exposure to inhalants. In studies using cats, repeated exposure to paint thinner produced hallucinations and convulsions and caused incoordination, catatonia, stereotyped, or continuously repeated, behavior, and an increase in overall behavioral activity—all of which could be related to changes in EEG.

Other Effects

Volatile organic solvents have toxic effects on various other parts of the body. One of the first areas to be damaged by inhalant abuse is the lining of the lungs, which can swell and make breathing difficult, even after exposure. Some solvents can produce painful swelling in and damage to the lining of the liver as well as burst blood vessels in the kidneys. Inflam-

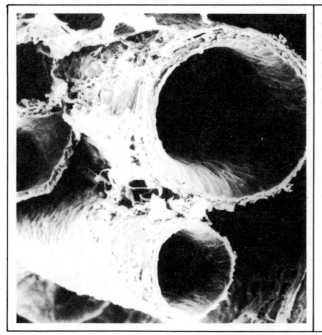

A microphotograph of tiny blood vessels in the human brain. Inhaling solvents breaks down delicate cell matter and can sometimes cause cerebral hemorrhaging.

mation and vascular (blood vessel) deformities are probably due to a decrease in the blood vessels' permeability, or the ability of materials to pass into and out of the vessels. Bone marrow can be damaged, resulting in a decrease in the production of both red and white blood cells and antibodies, which help to fight infection. The reproductive organs may also be affected adversely.

Inhaling solvents can also cause hemorrhages, or excessive bleeding, in various areas of the brain. Although changes in both the number and structure of brain cells have been noted, few reports indicate permanent damage. Therefore,

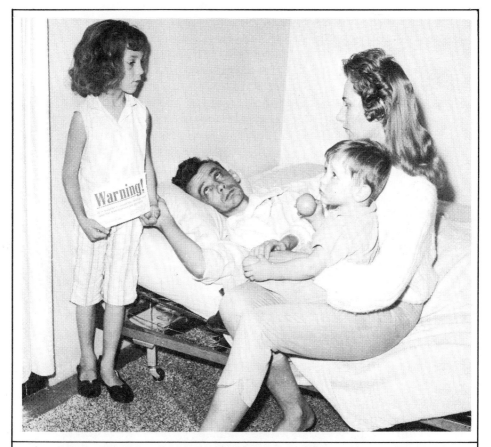

After being exposed to the poisonous fumes of mercury vapor, this family was quarantined and their home condemned because of fear that residual traces of the substance would spread.

the insomnia and depression often associated with chronic inhalant abuse are probably not due to brain damage.

Some of the earliest scientific studies focused on how exposure to toxic substances affects the normal functioning of the sensory system. Several incidents made it clear that this system is very sensitive to the effects of exposure. In the early 1950s Japanese industries began dumping waste into the Sea of Japan. Among the waste was methyl mercury, a naturally occurring form of the metal mercury. The methyl mercury was absorbed by plants, which were then eaten by fish. Because the human body does not rapidly break down methyl mercury, people who ate the fish began to accumulate increasing quantities of this chemical compound, which resulted in the destruction of certain cells in the retina of the eye and in reduced vision.

Today it is known that carbon disulfide gradually destroys some of the cells in the eye, creating a condition known as tunnel vision, characterized by a reduction of the visual field until only the area directly ahead is visible. Drinking methanol, or wood alcohol, rather than ethanol, frequently results in total blindness. Toluene, as well as other solvents, has been shown to destroy high frequency hearing.

In fact, the auditory, olfactory, cutaneous (relating to the skin), and gustatory (relating to the sense of taste) systems are all affected by abuse of inhalants. Testing a person for his or her sensory capability is thus one way to measure prior exposure to solvents. In addition, since sensory nerves are very similar to brain cells, it is very possible that the determination of sensory impairment also indicates some degree of brain damage.

Perhaps one of the most alarming cases of solvent-induced nervous system damage has been caused by the abuse of hexane. This substance, as well as some ketones, can cause a loss of sensation in the user's hands and feet. Though the effects of repeated low-level exposure can be reversed after several months of abstinence, some doses do cause permanent damage. In the 1930s a type of solvent known as tri-ortho-cresyl-phosphate was inadvertently included in a medicinal preparation known as "Jamaica ginger." Ingestion of this solvent by as many as 50,000 people resulted in their becoming paralyzed, a condition from which users either very slowly recovered or did not recover at all. Since this occurrence, there have been eight or nine other major outbreaks of tri-ortho-cresyl-phosphate poisonings.

Repeated exposure to ethanol can also affect the nervous system and cause a *senile dementia* (a condition of deteriorated mentality) known as Korsakoff's syndrome. This syndrome is characterized by *psychosis* (an emotional disorder whose symptoms include derangement of the personality and loss of contact with reality), disorientation, insomnia, memory loss, and hallucinations. Since it is possible that other inhalants act in a manner similar to ethanol, chronic abusers of other solvents may also be risking this same disease.

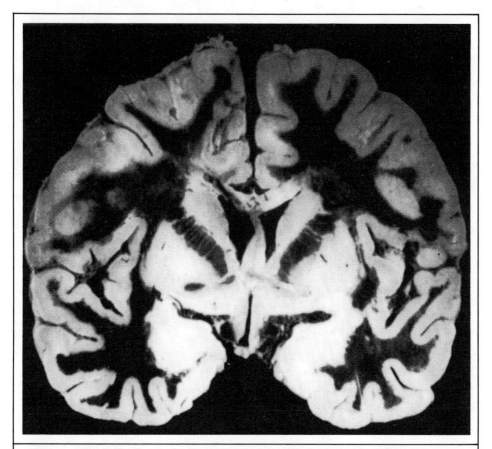

Cross section of a brain from a person who died of an alcoholic dementia that caused lesions, or holes, in the brain tissues. Frequent solvent inhalation has been known to cause similar symptoms.

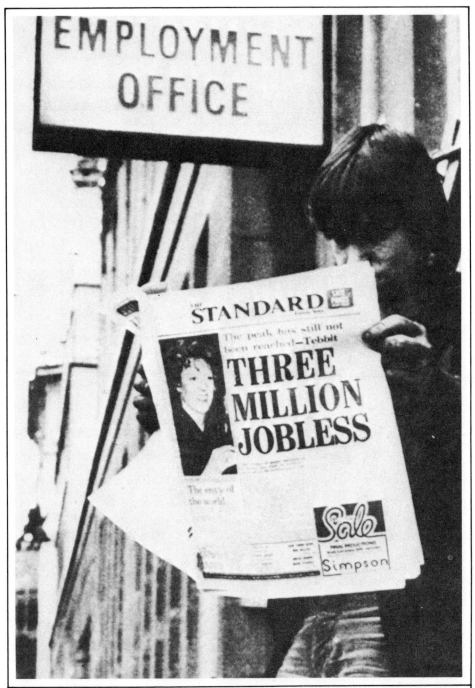

Headlines of a London newspaper cite recent unemployment statistics. For those without a job or money, the relatively cheap practice of glue and solvent sniffing is, unfortunately, often a misguided way to kill time.

CHAPTER 6

THE EPIDEMIOLOGY OF SOLVENT ABUSE

*E*pidemiology is the science that deals with the incidence, distribution, and control of disease in a population. The epidemiology of inhalants has been most concerned with determining the relationship between environment and those populations that are, or are likely to become, solvent abusers. Since not all people abuse solvents, it is quite possible that the practice is related to one or more factors in the abuser's environment. If these factors can be pinpointed, it is possible that they can be changed in a way that decreases the incidence of drug abuse.

In this type of research, scientists must be careful to consider all variables. For example, if it is found that solvent abuse is more prevalent in younger school-aged children, it must first be determined if this age group also uses other types of illicit drugs in high proportions before researchers can conclude that age is related to solvent use.

By using routine survey methods to question members of different groups, epidemiologists hope to discover patterns of drug abuse. Unfortunately, very few studies of this sort have focused on solvent abuse. Most of the available information comes from Mexico, where inhalant abuse was studied in two large cities, Mexico City and Districo Federale, and one small city, Queretaro. An additional study was done in Merida, the capital of Yucatan. Interestingly, some of the results of these surveys were very similar to those of a study completed in New York State.

In all of the studies, two factors were consistently related to solvent abuse: a person's sex and school performance. Gender was the most consistent variable. In the large Mexican cities, four times as many males as females were regular users; in the smaller Mexican city, three times as many males as females were regular users. In New York State, males were also more likely to abuse solvents. Poor school performance was also directly related to use of inhalants. In fact, a higher percentage of solvent abusers fail school than do their peers. The level of education was also found to be related to the extent of solvent abuse. Approximately three times as many regular users did not finish secondary school as those who did not use inhalants. One exception to this tendency, however, was in Mexico City, where there were no reports of individuals dropping out of school because of solvent use.

Although factors such as gender and poor school performance may be associated with solvent abuse, the extent to which each is either a cause or an effect is not clear. For example, although four times as many males as females use solvents, this does not mean that there is anything particular about being male that is directly related to becoming a solvent abuser. It is more likely that the behavioral patterns common to young males will bring them into contact with other solvent users, thereby increasing the opportunity to experiment with these drugs. People are typically introduced to drug abuse through social interactions. This simply means that a person will do what his or her friends are doing. Once the user breaks out of the pattern of social use and begins to inhale solvents when alone, he or she is likely to become a compulsive drug abuser.

With regard to school, poor performance could easily be interpreted as being an effect of the behavioral and/or health consequences of solvent exposure. However, failure in school may also reflect bad study habits that existed prior to involvement with inhalants. A sense of failure coupled with large amounts of free time could greatly increase the probability of using inhalants.

Another variable related to solvent abuse is the home situation. According to a New York State study, young people from broken homes are more likely to abuse solvents than their peers from more stable home environments. The lack of a well-structured family unit, therefore, appears to increase the influence of one's peers. However, because many solvent abusers do not come from broken homes, the home itself is not the major determinant of solvent abuse. In addition, few studies focusing on the relation between inhalants and home life have actually analyzed such factors as number of parents at home or the influence of siblings. Clearly, more accurate research is necessary.

Epidemiological studies have found that the average age of a solvent user is between 14 and 17 years. In the larger Mexican cities, less than 1% of the people older than 17 use inhalants on a regular basis ("regular use" is defined as at least once per day), though 1.3% of the 14- to 17-year-olds use inhalants regularly. The average age to start solvent abuse is 14 years. In the smaller cities, the percentage of solvent-

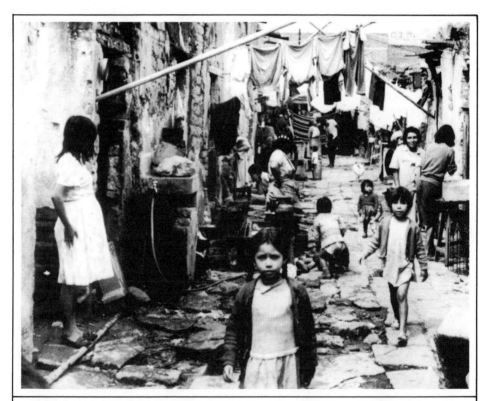

This slum area of Mexico City is an example of what sociologists have termed "a culture of poverty," complete with an established pattern of behavior, including solvent abuse as a standard means of intoxication.

using people between 12 and 18 years is higher (2.53%–4.23%) and the greatest rate of abuse is in individuals over 18 years old. In New York State more than 5% of the children in grades 7–12 have used solvents. Many of these solvent users cited peer pressure as the greatest influence on their decision to try inhalants.

In the larger suburbs of the Mexican cities, young people from the lower-income classes use solvents less than those from middle-income families. In Queretaro more people in the lower-income class (4.76%) use inhalants than those in the middle-income class (3.82%). In New York State the use of solvents is greater in young people with less educated parents and from poorer families. The influence of employment was considered only in the Districo Federale study. The results show that solvent abuse is more prominent among the unemployed. At least in this area it seems that the incidence of inhalant abuse increases with age and is greater among people of lower classes.

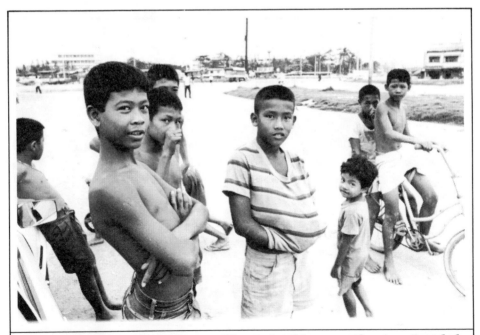

A group of youths, some of them sniffing paint thinner, gather in a Bangkok ghetto. Abusers of addictive drugs are often youngsters—the boy driving the bicycle is a former heroin addict: he is 14 years old.

From the studies cited above, certain patterns become evident. In the Mexican studies, both the incidence of abuse and the age of the abuser decrease as the population becomes more urban. In the New York study, the patterns of use are similar. Rural parts of the state have a greater number of solvent abusers than the suburbs of New York City, while the suburbs have more abusers than the city itself. In addition, solvent abuse seems to be more popular in smaller cities (and perhaps in the country), and poor males probably abuse solvents for longer periods of time.

Polydrug Use

Some of these studies also asked questions about the use of other drugs. Of all of the drugs abused, including heroin and the hallucinogens, only marijuana was used more than solvents. Though alcohol use was not included in these studies, it could be an important factor in solvent abuse. Alcohol abusers may resort to using inhalants when their preferred drug is not available.

In addition to the physical, psychological, sociological, and economic influences, other factors can come into play. A significant factor in solvent abuse is availability of the substance. Because solvents are inexpensive and easy to find, they appeal to people who may have difficulty finding other mind-altering drugs and/or who are too poor to afford alcohol and other more expensive drugs.

In the 1980s *polydrug use*, or the abuse of many drugs, has emerged as a prominent aspect of the drug abuser's lifestyle. With the possible exception of many alcohol and marijuana users, most drug users abuse several substances. Of all the solvent users questioned, only 24% used solvents only. The most common second drug of abuse is alcohol. In fact, only 22% of the polydrug users ingest inhalants and just one other drug—10% use at least two other substances, 11% use at least three, 16% use at least four, and 17% use five or more. Obviously, the majority of solvent users are polydrug users. Among inhalant users, 98% use alcohol, 75% use marijuana, 50% use stimulants and depressants, and 50% use hallucinogens and opiates.

Interestingly, solvent use often precedes the use of all other drugs. For polydrug users, solvents emerged as the first substance abused in 53% of the cases; in 34% of the cases, solvents were the second substance used. This finding may suggest that the abuse of inhalants does, in fact, lead to the use of many drugs.

The Typical Inhalant Abuser

Though it is difficult to predict who will use inhalants, researchers have created the profile of the typical abuser. One case study describes a woman who closely fits the picture. Twenty-three years old and with a high school education and a 10-year history of drug abuse, this woman was physically dependent on aerosol spray paints. For two years she sniffed, paints, plastic enamels, and paint thinners daily for up to five hours. She would place a paint-saturated cloth in her mouth and inhale the vapors, a practice that kept her continuously intoxicated. Typically, the paint contained toluene.

The woman's parents, both alcoholics, were separated. Her social life was very limited, and her own marriage had ended in separation. She had been arrested at least 30 times, once for assaulting a policeman, and on two occasions the woman had become so depressed that she had taken drugs in an attempt to commit suicide.

When she was admitted to the hospital, she complained of chronic muscular pain and a loss of sensation in her hands and feet. However, a routine physical examination revealed no sensory or neuromuscular problems. Though toxicology tests failed to detect the presence of any drugs, the results of further tests suggested the possibility of a developing muscular abnormality. Previously, she had been hospitalized for acute organic brain syndrome, or brain damage, a common diagnosis given to solvent abusers. After 16 days of treatment the patient was discharged.

Toxicity in the Workplace

Though many young solvent abusers develop their practice through peer influence, at least one group of drug users may have been inadvertently exposed and subsequently addicted to inhalants. Factory and shop workers are often exposed to volatile organic solvents while using equipment such as degreasing machines and paint sprayers. When ventilation is not adequate, concentrations often reach levels sufficient to produce behavioral effects. There are several accounts of degreasing-machine operators who first became attracted to the smell of trichloroethylene at work and later went on to abuse the solvent at home.

Socioeconomic factors contribute to this problem. People who are poor or whose training or education does not allow them to find other work may be more willing to work under adverse situations. In addition, the fear of losing one's job may make a person less apt to complain when solvent concentrations rise above toxic levels. The most effective way to combat this situation is to determine and enforce safe levels of toxic substances at the workplace. The regulations may originate at the level of the federal government, but their enforcement must include cooperation by both the workers and the management.

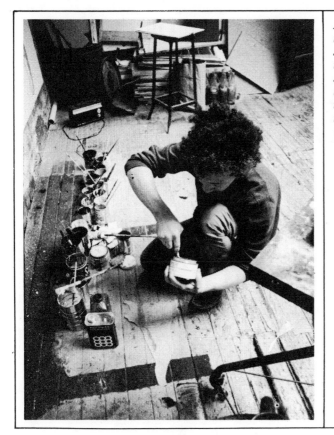

An artist mixes paint thinner in his studio. Solvents such as thinners and glue are so common in daily life that education about the dire hazards of their abuse is of the utmost importance.

Establishing Safe Solvent Levels

The question of which solvent levels are safe and can be tolerated without incident and which are toxic can be approached from various angles. One approach is to find the lethal dose, or LD 50, by administering different solvent concentrations to experimental animals to determine the dose that kills 50% of the subjects, and then reducing this figure by a factor of at least 1000. This method suffers because the variability in the animals' responses may be large—even though 50% of the animals may have died at a certain concentration, a few may have died at concentrations of even 100 times less. This means that more sensitive individuals will be at risk at solvent levels that are supposedly safe for

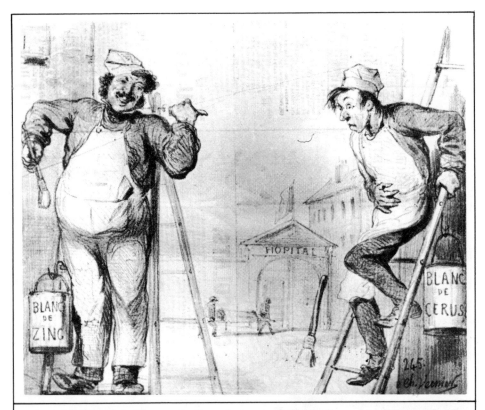

An old lithograph illustrates the advantages of zinc-based paint over lead-based paint, the fumes of which could cause lead poisoning.

others. In addition, it is often incorrect to assume that data collected from animals can be readily and/or accurately applied to humans.

Another approach is to set the acceptable concentration based on the lowest level that will produce any behavioral, cardiovascular, electrophysiological (relating to the electrical aspects of the body's functions), cytological (pertaining to the cells), or other effects. This method is especially well suited for those solvents that produce behavioral effects at lower concentrations. However, to accurately assess all the effects of the solvents, this approach requires large and expensive testing programs. Unfortunately, current acceptable limits are generally based on the assessment of only one or two effects.

Both of these approaches establish for each particular solvent a Threshold Limit Value, a Time Weighted Average, or a Maximum Allowable Concentration, and this amount is

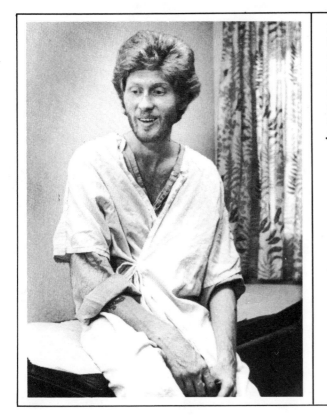

This Kansas City man was rescued from a sewer after he had blacked out while sniffing glue in a manhole. He fell 20 feet down the shaft and was lost underground for 24 hours.

not to be exceeded in the industrial setting. For example, the current Threshold Limit Value for toluene is 100 ppm (parts per million). Though this is only 3 to 4 times lower than concentrations that have produced behavioral effects, if this level were never exceeded, workers exposed to toluene at their workplaces would probably not become solvent abusers.

Scientists are only beginning to formulate a complete picture of the environment that fosters the dangerous practice of inhalant abuse. It would be helpful to be able to identify the individual who is abusing solvents in school or at the workplace, but such attempts might involve intruding upon personal freedoms. Nonetheless, it is clear that these efforts would benefit both the individual and society.

One way to detect small quantities of a drug or the drug's metabolites is to test the blood or urine. This method has been widely and successfully used to measure alcohol concentrations of automobile drivers. In addition, the U.S. Army employed similar tests for detecting drugs in soldiers returning from Vietnam, where drug use was widespread. Today there are private employers who screen their workers for drugs such as marijuana. Similar tests could be developed that would be sensitive to solvents. Though these substances are rapidly eliminated from the body, it is possible that the metabolites could be detected.

The intoxicated individual can be identified by several characteristics. Some of these are the odor of the solvent on the breath, disorientation, incoordination, stupor, and slurred speech. However, these effects often disappear soon after inhalation. Additional indications of abuse are signs of malnutrition and a general disregard for personal appearance.

Once the solvent abuser has been identified, the counselor, co-worker, parent, or teacher must know how to handle the problem. Many drug-treatment programs are familiar with solvent abuse and can help compulsive abusers restructure their lives to decrease the probability of relapse once inhalant use has stopped. Although no reliable figures are available, the rate of relapse to solvent abuse (excluding alcohol) appears to be low. In chronic cases of solvent abuse, the drug user may be counseled to attend social support groups such as Alcoholics Anonymous (AA). For alcohol abusers, who in general have a very high relapse rate, organizations such as

AA provide one of the best ways to gain self-control over drug abuse.

Other alternatives are more drastic. Researchers working with animals have experimented with ways in which punishment can be used to decrease or eliminate drug-seeking behavior. However, these methods generally are not successful when applied to humans because the punishment is most effective only in the environment in which it was delivered. Once outside of that environment the individual again seeks the drug. As mentioned earlier, Antabuse has been used with some success with alcoholics. In effect, this substance, which works in any environment, punishes a person every time he or she consumes alcohol. The success of this method depends upon continuous use of Antabuse or the ability to refrain from drinking once this medication is stopped. Unfortunately, agents that produce negative effects when in the presence of other solvents have not yet been developed.

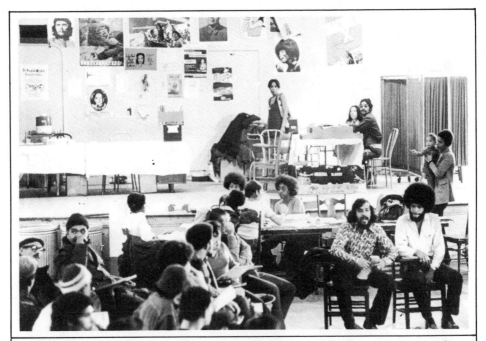

People with drug problems share their thoughts and feelings at a counseling session. In many cases such meetings help addicts to understand the reasons why they resorted to drugs in the first place.

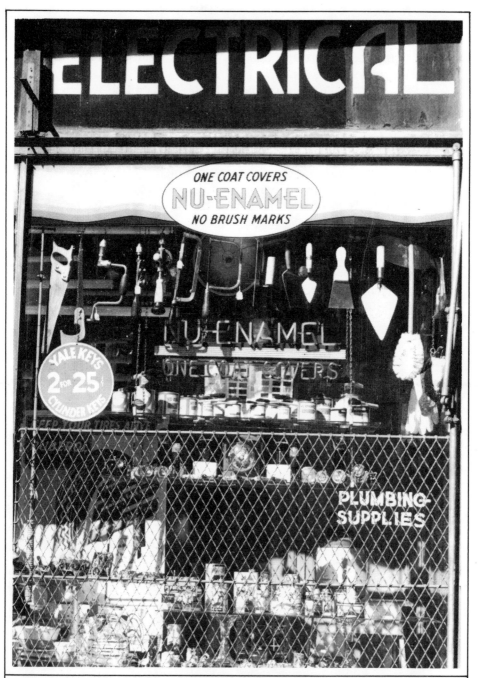

Volatile organic solvents are legally available from a wide variety of sources. Inhaling these solvents has been proven to be seriously damaging to one's health, often causing widespread permanent damage to the mind and body of the abuser.

CHAPTER 7

INHALANTS AND THE LAW

Most drugs are controlled by the Drug Enforcement Administration, which lists each substance under one of five schedules. A drug's placement in a schedule determines its availability for both medical and nonmedical applications as well as the penalty for its illegal use. For example, drugs that have the greatest abuse potential and no accepted medical use, such as heroin and LSD, are in Schedule I. Drugs with the least abuse potential and well-established medical use are in Schedule V. Interestingly, most inhalants are not in any schedule.

A person of any age can purchase substances such as toluene, acetone, and octane without prescription or license from chemical supply stores, industrial suppliers, and even drug stores. Many of these inhalants can also be found in common household or industrial mixtures that are readily available. Just a few solvents, such as amyl nitrite, are controlled and dispensed by prescription only. Though some agents, such as nitrous oxide, halothane, and ethyl alcohol, may be more difficult to obtain in pure forms, they can still be found in places such as warehouses, clinics, or schools, where, unfortunately, the substances are not closely watched. Thus, despite their obvious danger to an individual's health, volatile organic solvents are not as difficult to find as chemically manufactured drugs such as amphetamines and barbiturates. In addition, inhalants are considerably less expensive than drugs such as alcohol and marijuana.

Some inhalants should be scheduled, but their need in legitimate industrial processes makes this very difficult. However, their purchase could be monitored and their levels could be checked in areas where larger than normal levels of solvents are being used. In the past, restrictions have not been very successful because most of the solvents are very easy to produce and/or find. More recently, several alternative approaches have been suggested.

Solving the Problem of Solvent Abuse

The most popular approach has been to try to decrease the solvents' abuse potential by adding irritants or other chemicals. For example, irritants have been added to mixtures, such as model airplane glue, so that when they are inhaled they cause choking and tearing. Similarly, a substance has been added to ethyl alcohol that "denatures" the alcohol and thus makes it essentially undrinkable.

Another solution is to change the composition of products that include solvents with abuse potential. This measure would force manufacturers to find suitable substitutes for the solvent. Unfortunately, this is not an easy or inexpensive task and manufacturers are reluctant to choose it as a solution.

Though limiting sales and/or access would seem to be a good way to curb abuse, this is not very practical because the legal process often takes longer than the discovery pro-

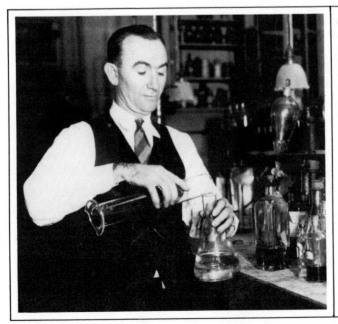

A chemist in the 1920s grimaces as he works with a denaturant, a substance added to some solvents as an irritant intended to discourage abuse.

cess for finding suitable alternatives. This guarantees that the abuser will probably not be denied access to at least some abusable substances.

The last and most frequently mentioned solution involves community action. This, however, requires a well-educated public and a commitment to change. Because, as mentioned earlier, few people are aware of the extent of the solvent abuse problem, strong programs focusing on the recognition and treatment of solvent abuse must be developed. Most importantly, the nature of drug abuse must be understood.

Solvent abuse is very similar to the abuse of any other drug or to other forms of obsessive behavior, such as excessive eating and exercising. Given the great risk associated with inhalant abuse, it would appear that the best way to deal with this problem is to educate the public to the dangers of solvent use and to provide suitable alternatives for the abuser. An incomplete understanding of the nature of compulsive behavior decreases community commitment and thus makes finding suitable alternatives difficult. This is especially a problem in communities in which solvent use is more socially acceptable.

Volatile organic solvents constitute a threat to the health and well being of society. They have a variety of adverse health effects and have pronounced abuse potential. Abuse of inhalants is more harmful to the individual and society than the abuse of many other drugs, and yet less effort has been made to curb such practices. There is also sufficient evidence to suggest that inhalant abuse is one of the easiest, least expensive, and perhaps most pervasive means of getting involved in the habit of drug abuse. Special efforts should be made to educate the public about the dangers and symptoms of, and the alternatives to, volatile solvent abuse.

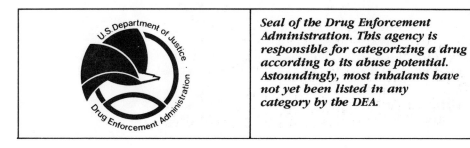

Seal of the Drug Enforcement Administration. This agency is responsible for categorizing a drug according to its abuse potential. Astoundingly, most inhalants have not yet been listed in any category by the DEA.

APPENDIX

STATE AGENCIES
FOR THE PREVENTION AND TREATMENT
OF DRUG ABUSE

ALABAMA
Department of Mental Health
Division of Mental Illness and
  Substance Abuse Community
  Programs
200 Interstate Park Drive
P.O. Box 3710
Montgomery, AL 36193
(205) 271-9253

ALASKA
Department of Health and Social
  Services
Office of Alcoholism and Drug
  Abuse
Pouch H-05-F
Juneau, AK 99811
(907) 586-6201

ARIZONA
Department of Health Services
Division of Behavioral Health
  Services
Bureau of Community Services
Alcohol Abuse and Alcoholism
  Section
2500 East Van Buren
Phoenix, AZ 85008
(602) 255-1238

Department of Health Services
Division of Behavioral Health
  Services
Bureau of Community Services
Drug Abuse Section
2500 East Van Buren
Phoenix, AZ 85008
(602) 255-1240

ARKANSAS
Department of Human Services
Office on Alcohol and Drug Abuse
  Prevention
1515 West 7th Avenue
Suite 310
Little Rock, AR 72202
(501) 371-2603

CALIFORNIA
Department of Alcohol and Drug
  Abuse
111 Capitol Mall
Sacramento, CA 95814
(916) 445-1940

COLORADO
Department of Health
Alcohol and Drug Abuse Division
4210 East 11th Avenue
Denver, CO 80220
(303) 320-6137

CONNECTICUT
Alcohol and Drug Abuse
  Commission
999 Asylum Avenue
3rd Floor
Hartford, CT 06105
(203) 566-4145

DELAWARE
Division of Mental Health
Bureau of Alcoholism and Drug
  Abuse
1901 North Dupont Highway
Newcastle, DE 19720
(302) 421-6101

DISTRICT OF COLUMBIA
Department of Human Services
Office of Health Planning and
  Development
601 Indiana Avenue, NW
Suite 500
Washington, D.C. 20004
(202) 724-5641

FLORIDA
Department of Health and
  Rehabilitative Services
Alcoholic Rehabilitation Program
1317 Winewood Boulevard
Room 187A
Tallahassee, FL 32301
(904) 488-0396

Department of Health and
  Rehabilitative Services
Drug Abuse Program
1317 Winewood Boulevard
Building 6, Room 155
Tallahassee, FL 32301
(904) 488-0900

GEORGIA
Department of Human Resources
Division of Mental Health and
  Mental Retardation
Alcohol and Drug Section
618 Ponce De Leon Avenue, NE
Atlanta, GA 30365-2101
(404) 894-4785

HAWAII
Department of Health
Mental Health Division
Alcohol and Drug Abuse Branch
1250 Punch Bowl Street
P.O. Box 3378
Honolulu, HI 96801
(808) 548-4280

IDAHO
Department of Health and Welfare
Bureau of Preventive Medicine
Substance Abuse Section
450 West State
Boise, ID 83720
(208) 334-4368

ILLINOIS
Department of Mental Health and
  Developmental Disabilities
Division of Alcoholism
160 North La Salle Street
Room 1500
Chicago, IL 60601
(312) 793-2907

Illinois Dangerous Drugs
  Commission
300 North State Street
Suite 1500
Chicago, IL 60610
(312) 822-9860

INDIANA
Department of Mental Health
Division of Addiction Services
429 North Pennsylvania Street
Indianapolis, IN 46204
(317) 232-7816

IOWA
Department of Substance Abuse
505 5th Avenue
Insurance Exchange Building
Suite 202
Des Moines, IA 50319
(515) 281-3641

KANSAS
Department of Social Rehabilitation
Alcohol and Drug Abuse Services
2700 West 6th Street
Biddle Building
Topeka, KS 66606
(913) 296-3925

KENTUCKY
Cabinet for Human Resources
Department of Health Services
Substance Abuse Branch
275 East Main Street
Frankfort, KY 40601
(502) 564-2880

LOUISIANA
Department of Health and Human
    Resources
Office of Mental Health and
    Substance Abuse
655 North 5th Street
P.O. Box 4049
Baton Rouge, LA 70821
(504) 342-2565

MAINE
Department of Human Services
Office of Alcoholism and Drug
    Abuse Prevention
Bureau of Rehabilitation
32 Winthrop Street
Augusta, ME 04330
(207) 289-2781

MARYLAND
Alcoholism Control Administration
201 West Preston Street
Fourth Floor
Baltimore, MD 21201
(301) 383-2977

State Health Department
Drug Abuse Administration
201 West Preston Street
Baltimore, MD 21201
(301) 383-3312

MASSACHUSETTS
Department of Public Health
Division of Alcoholism
755 Boylston Street
Sixth Floor
Boston, MA 02116
(617) 727-1960

Department of Public Health
Division of Drug Rehabilitation
600 Washington Street
Boston, MA 02114
(617) 727-8617

MICHIGAN
Department of Public Health
Office of Substance Abuse Services
3500 North Logan Street
P.O. Box 30035
Lansing, MI 48909
(517) 373-8603

MINNESOTA
Department of Public Welfare
Chemical Dependency Program
    Division
Centennial Building
658 Cedar Street
4th Floor
Saint Paul, MN 55155
(612) 296-4614

MISSISSIPPI
Department of Mental Health
Division of Alcohol and Drug Abuse
1102 Robert E. Lee Building
Jackson, MS 39201
(601) 359-1297

MISSOURI
Department of Mental Health
Division of Alcoholism and Drug
    Abuse
2002 Missouri Boulevard
P.O. Box 687
Jefferson City, MO 65102
(314) 751-4942

MONTANA
Department of Institutions
Alcohol and Drug Abuse Division
1539 11th Avenue
Helena, MT 59620
(406) 449-2827

NEBRASKA
Department of Public Institutions
Division of Alcoholism and Drug Abuse
801 West Van Dorn Street
P.O. Box 94728
Lincoln, NB 68509
(402) 471-2851, Ext. 415

NEVADA
Department of Human Resources
Bureau of Alcohol and Drug Abuse
505 East King Street
Carson City, NV 89710
(702) 885-4790

NEW HAMPSHIRE
Department of Health and Welfare
Office of Alcohol and Drug Abuse
   Prevention
Hazen Drive
Health and Welfare Building
Concord, NH 03301
(603) 271-4627

NEW JERSEY
Department of Health
Division of Alcoholism
129 East Hanover Street CN 362
Trenton, NJ 08625
(609) 292-8949

Department of Health
Division of Narcotic and Drug Abuse
   Control
129 East Hanover Street CN 362
Trenton, NJ 08625
(609) 292-8949

NEW MEXICO
Health and Environment Department
Behavioral Services Division
Substance Abuse Bureau
725 Saint Michaels Drive
P.O. Box 968
Santa Fe, NM 87503
(505) 984-0020, Ext. 304

NEW YORK
Division of Alcoholism and Alcohol
   Abuse
194 Washington Avenue
Albany, NY 12210
(518) 474-5417

Division of Substance Abuse
   Services
Executive Park South
Box 8200
Albany, NY 12203
(518) 457-7629

NORTH CAROLINA
Department of Human Resources
Division of Mental Health, Mental
   Retardation and Substance Abuse
   Services
Alcohol and Drug Abuse Services
325 North Salisbury Street
Albemarle Building
Raleigh, NC 27611
(919) 733-4670

NORTH DAKOTA
Department of Human Services
Division of Alcoholism and Drug
   Abuse
State Capitol Building
Bismarck, ND 58505
(701) 224-2767

OHIO
Department of Health
Division of Alcoholism
246 North High Street
P.O. Box 118
Columbus, OH 43216
(614) 466-3543

Department of Mental Health
Bureau of Drug Abuse
65 South Front Street
Columbus, OH 43215
(614) 466-9023

OKLAHOMA
Department of Mental Health
Alcohol and Drug Programs
4545 North Lincoln Boulevard
Suite 100 East Terrace
P.O. Box 53277
Oklahoma City, OK 73152
(405) 521-0044

OREGON
Department of Human Resources
Mental Health Division
Office of Programs for Alcohol and
    Drug Problems
2575 Bittern Street, NE
Salem, OR 97310
(503) 378-2163

PENNSYLVANIA
Department of Health
Office of Drug and Alcohol
    Programs
Commonwealth and Forster Avenues
Health and Welfare Building
P.O. Box 90
Harrisburg, PA 17108
(717) 787-9857

RHODE ISLAND
Department of Mental Health,
    Mental Retardation and Hospitals
Division of Substance Abuse
Substance Abuse Administration
    Building
Cranston, RI 02920
(401) 464-2091

SOUTH CAROLINA
Commission on Alcohol and Drug
    Abuse
3700 Forest Drive
Columbia, SC 29204
(803) 758-2521

SOUTH DAKOTA
Department of Health
Division of Alcohol and Drug Abuse
523 East Capitol, Joe Foss Building
Pierre, SD 57501
(605) 773-4806

TENNESSEE
Department of Mental Health and
    Mental Retardation
Alcohol and Drug Abuse Services
505 Deaderick Street
James K. Polk Building, Fourth Floor
Nashville, TN 37219
(615) 741-1921

TEXAS
Commission on Alcoholism
809 Sam Houston State Office Building
Austin, TX 78701
(512) 475-2577

Department of Community Affairs
Drug Abuse Prevention Division
2015 South Interstate Highway 35
P.O. Box 13166
Austin, TX 78711
(512) 443-4100

UTAH
Department of Social Services
Division of Alcoholism and Drugs
150 West North Temple
Suite 350
P.O. Box 2500
Salt Lake City, UT 84110
(801) 533-6532

VERMONT
Agency of Human Services
Department of Social and
    Rehabilitation Services
Alcohol and Drug Abuse Division
103 South Main Street
Waterbury, VT 05676
(802) 241-2170

VIRGINIA
Department of Mental Health and
  Mental Retardation
Division of Substance Abuse
109 Governor Street
P.O. Box 1797
Richmond, VA 23214
(804) 786-5313

WASHINGTON
Department of Social and Health
  Service
Bureau of Alcohol and Substance
  Abuse
Office Building—44 W
Olympia, WA 98504
(206) 753-5866

WEST VIRGINIA
Department of Health
Office of Behavioral Health Services
Division on Alcoholism and Drug
  Abuse
1800 Washington Street East
Building 3 Room 451
Charleston, WV 25305
(304) 348-2276

WISCONSIN
Department of Health and Social
  Services
Division of Community Services
Bureau of Community Programs
Alcohol and Other Drug Abuse
  Program Office
1 West Wilson Street
P.O. Box 7851
Madison, WI 53707
(608) 266-2717

WYOMING
Alcohol and Drug Abuse Programs
Hathaway Building
Cheyenne, WY 82002
(307) 777-7115, Ext. 7118

GUAM
Mental Health & Substance Abuse
  Agency
P.O. Box 20999
Guam 96921

PUERTO RICO
Department of Addiction Control
  Services
Alcohol Abuse Programs
P.O. Box B-Y Rio Piedras Station
Rio Piedras, PR 00928
(809) 763-5014

Department of Addiction Control
  Services
Drug Abuse Programs
P.O. Box B-Y Rio Piedras Station
Rio Piedras, PR 00928
(809) 764-8140

VIRGIN ISLANDS
Division of Mental Health,
  Alcoholism & Drug Dependency
  Services
P.O. Box 7329
Saint Thomas, Virgin Islands 00801
(809) 774-7265

AMERICAN SAMOA
LBJ Tropical Medical Center
Department of Mental Health Clinic
Pago Pago, American Samoa 96799

TRUST TERRITORIES
Director of Health Services
Office of the High Commissioner
Saipan, Trust Territories 96950

Further Reading

Brecher, Edward M., and the editors of *Consumer Reports. Licit and Illicit Drugs, The Consumer Union Report on Narcotics, Stimulants, Depressants, Inhalants, Hallucinogens, and Marijuana—Including Caffeine, Nicotine, & Alcohol.* Mount Vernon, New York: Consumers Union, 1972.

Cohen, S. "Inhalant Abuse: An Overview of the Problem," in *Review of Inhalants: Euphoria to Dysfunction.* NIDA Monograph, no. 15. Rockville, Maryland: U.S. Government Printing Office, 1977.

Comstock, E.G. and Comstock, B.S. "Medical Evaluation of Inhalant Abusers," in *Review of Inhalants: Euphoria to Dysfunction.* NIDA Monograph, no. 15. Rockville, Maryland: U.S. Government Printing Office, 1977.

Glowa, John R. "The Behavioral Effects of Volatile Organic Solvents," in Balster, R.L. and Seiden, L.S., eds. *Behavioral Pharmacology: A Generation of Progress.* New York: Alan Liss, 1985.

Nagle, David R. "Anesthetic Addiction and Drunkenness," in *International Journal of the Addictions*, vol. 3, 1968.

Patty, Frank A. *Industrial Hygiene and Toxicology*, vol. II. New York: John Wiley & Sons, 1963.

Wolman, H. and Smith, T.C. "Uptake, Distribution, Elimination, and Administration of Inhalational Anesthetics," in Goodman, L.S. and Gilman, A., eds. *The Pharmacological Basis of Therapeutics.* New York: Macmillan, 1975.

Wood, R.W. "Stimulus Properties of Inhaled Substances: An Update," in Mitchell, C.L. *Nervous System Toxicology.* New York: Raven Press, 1982.

Glossary

alcohol   a class of organic compounds that includes methyl alcohol, ethyl alcohol, and isopropyl alcohol and is composed of hydrogen (H), carbon (C), and one or more hydroxyl (oxygen and hydrogen, or OH) groups

alipathic hydrocarbon   a type of molecule composed only of straight chains of carbon atoms attached to hydrogen atoms, e.g., octane, heptane, and hexane

anoxia   a deficiency of oxygen resulting from either an anemic condition, characterized by a deficiency in the oxygen-carrying abilities of the blood, or diminished oxygen in the blood in the arteries, caused by reduced oxygen supply, respiratory obstruction, decreased surface area in the lungs (as in pneumonia), or inadequate breathing

antagonist   a substance that blocks or counteracts the action of another substance

anticonvulsant   a substance that prevents or relieves convulsions

aromatic hydrocarbon   a type of molecule composed of a central ring of carbon atoms to which hydrogen atoms are attached, e.g., benzene and toluene

axon   the part of the neuron along which the nerve impulse travels away from the cell body

barbiturate   a drug that causes depression of the central nervous system, generally used to reduce anxiety or to induce euphoria

behavioral toxicity   the extent, quality, or degree of being harmful to normal behavioral functioning

carcinogen   an agent capable of producing or promoting cancer

chloroform   a heavy, colorless, and liquid halogenated hydrocarbon that was once used to produce anesthesia

cocaine   the primary psychoactive ingredient in the coca plant and a behavioral stimulant

concentration   the proportion of one substance in another substance, often measured in parts per million (ppm) or weight per volume (milligrams per liter, or mg/l)

conditioned aversion   an aversion to a substance or aspect of the environment developed through pairing with an unpleasant experience such as illness or pain

delerium tremens   a psychological disorder, involving visual and auditory hallucinations, found in habitual and excessive users of alcohol

dendrite   the hairlike structure which protrudes from the neural cell body on which receptor sites are located

discriminative stimulus   something that acts as a cue to certain behaviors; for example, the smell of a solvent may make a solvent user more likely to engage in a specific set of behaviors

embryotoxic   capable of terminating pregnancy

epidemiology   a science that deals with the incidence, distribution, and control of disease in a population

ether   an organic compound composed of oxygen, carbon, and hydrogen such as diethyl ether ($C_4H_{10}O$), the form used to produce anesthesia

fermentation   a chemical process by which yeast consumes sugars, such as those in fruits, and produces effervescence and alcohol

formaldehyde   a colorless, pungent, and irritant gas (CHOH) used as a preservative and a disinfectant

free-base cocaine   the cocaine alkaloid, or base, which results when the hydrochloride is removed from cocaine hydrochloride, a common form of the drug

hallucinogen   a drug that produces sensory impressions that have no basis in reality

halogenated hydrocarbon   a compound, such as chloroform, trichloroethylene, or carbon tetrachloride, composed of carbon, hydrogen, and chlorine, bromine, iodine, or fluorine

hemorrhage   abnormal internal or external discharge of blood

ketone   a compound, such as acetone, that contains a carbonyl group (CO, or a carbon atom and an oxygen atom connected by a double bond)

lipophilic   absorbing or having an affinity for fat

marijuana   the leaves, flowers, buds, and/or branches of the hemp plant *Cannabis sativa* or *Cannabis indica* that contains cannabinoids, a group of intoxicating drugs

metabolism   the chemical changes in the living cell by which energy is provided for the vital processes and activities and by which new material is assimilated to repair cell structures; or, the process that uses enzymes to convert one substance into compounds that can be easily eliminated from the body

methaqualone 2-methyl-3-0-tolyl-4(3H)-quinazolinone; a white, bitter-tasting, crystalline powder with sedative/hypnotic effects; frequently known by the trade name Quaalude

neurotransmitter a chemical that travels from the axon of one neuron, across the synaptic gap, and to the receptor site on the dendrite of an adjacent neuron, thus allowing communication between neural cells

nicotine a volatile and highly poisonous stimulant naturally occurring in the tobacco plant

opiate a compound from the milky juice of the poppy plant *Papaver somniferum*, including opium, morphine, codeine, and their derivatives, such as heroin

organic pertaining to or derived from substances that contain carbon and hydrogen

paranoia a mental condition characterized by suspiciousness, fear, delusions, and, in extreme cases, hallucinations

PCP phencyclidine; a frequently abused synthetic anesthetic that in low doses produces mild euphoria and stimulation; in higher doses slurred speech, incoordination, and rapid thought process; in even higher doses immobility without loss of consciousness, and finally convulsions, coma, and death

pentobarbital a short-acting barbiturate

pharmacokinetics study of the metabolism and action of drugs, particularly absorption time, duration of action, distribution throughout the body, and elimination

psychoactive altering mood and/or behavior

psychosis a behavioral disorder characterized by a loss of contact with commonly perceived reality and symptoms such as delusions, hallucinations, and emotional and cognitive breakdown

reinforcing having the ability to maintain or increase the incidence or rate of a behavior

sedative-hypnotic drug a drug that produces a general depressant effect on the nervous system, such as relaxation, relief from anxiety, and sleep

solvent an agent, such as water, alcohol, or ether, that can dissolve another agent and form a solution

synapse   the microscopic gap between the axon and dendrite of two adjacent neurons in which neurotransmitters travel

synthesize   to form a complex substance from simpler elements or compounds

teratological effects   adverse effects caused by an agent on a developing fetus

tolerance   a decrease of susceptibility to the effects of a drug due to its continued administration, resulting in the user's need to increase the drug dosage in order to achieve the effects experienced previously

toluene   the aromatic hydrocarbon $C_6H_5CH_3$ which is a volatile solvent used in many industrial products such as glue and often abused as an inhalant

toxic   causing temporary or permanent damage to cells or organ systems of the body

trichloroethylene   the halogenated hydrocarbon CCl_2CHCl which is a volatile liquid with analgesic and anesthetic actions and which is sometimes abused as an inhalant

vapor pressure   the pressure exerted by a vapor that is in equilibrium with a solid or gas; an indication of the tendency of a substance to leave the liquid phase and enter the gas phase

volatile   characterized by the tendency to rapidly change from a liquid to a vapor

Index